The Cancer Problem

A Critical Analysis and Modern Synthesis

The Cancer Problem

A Critical Analysis and Modern Synthesis

Armin C. Braun

Columbia University Press
New York and London
1969

Armin C. Braun is Professor and Head of the Laboratory of Plant
Biology at The Rockefeller University in New York.

Copyright © 1969 Columbia University Press
Standard Book Number: 231-02938-1
Library of Congress Catalog Card Number: 77-90432
Printed in the United States of America

PREFACE

This book was born of a desire by the author to learn whether certain fundamental principles and concepts, which are so clearly illustrated in plant tumor systems, are applicable and might thus serve to provide insight into the basic cellular mechanisms that underlie neoplastic growth generally. The discussion that follows presents a point of view that has evolved during a lifetime of study of the plant tumor systems. The concepts upon which this point of view is based, and for which no originality is claimed, will be discussed against a background of our present understanding of the cancer problem. The word *cancer* is used here broadly, as it is often used by the experimentalist who is interested in the nature of the malignant process, rather than in the more restricted sense used by the surgeon or by the pathologist to designate malignancies of epithelial origin.

Since this book is essentially conceptual in nature and its purpose is to develop principles, no attempt has been made nor would it seem possible for any one person to review all of the pertinent literature in an area of scientific endeavor as vast as that covered here. Every effort has, nevertheless, been made to document, insofar as that is now possible, the main theme of this book, which states that the tumor problem is basically a problem of anomalous differentiation and that the fundamental cellular mechanisms underlying tumorigenesis are similar in principle to those involved in normal cellular differentiation. For that reason certain sections of this book are devoted to normal rather than abnormal aspects of growth and development. Because the discussion that follows is concerned with an understanding of the basic cellular mechanisms underlying tumorigenesis, certain large but important areas of cancer research such as chemotherapy and tumor immunology are touched upon only very briefly or not at all.

A book of this type is in a very real sense a cooperative effort and I am indeed grateful and owe so much to Miss Ella Jeanne Ross for her dedication, patience, and long hours of work in attempting to bring a semblance of order out of the often shapeless mass of manuscript and references that were submitted to her. I am also most grateful to Dr. James S. Henderson for reading and commenting on the first chapter as well as for critical discussions dealing with certain aspects of the animal tumor problem, to Dr. Antoine Simard for reading the second chapter, to Dr. Bernice Grafstein for helpful suggestions and comments concerning the fifth chapter, and to Dr. Samuel Balk for reading the entire manuscript before it was submitted to the publisher. To my colleague and research associate Dr. Henry N. Wood as well as to that inspiring group of young enthusiasts, the students in my laboratory, Dr. Balk, Mr. Carl V. Lundeen, Mr. Frederick Meins, Jr., and Mr. Eric S. Weinberg, who were helpful in so many ways, I owe a deep debt of thanks. I should also like to thank Dr. Roy E. Albert, Dr. James S. Henderson, Dr. Ian Macpherson, Dr. G. Barry Pierce, Jr., Dr. William J. Robbins, and Dr. Folke Skoog for kindly making available to the author original prints for use in this book.

I am, in addition, most grateful to the granting agencies—the American Cancer Society, Inc., the National Cancer Institute of the U. S. Public Health Service, and the National Science Foundation—for patiently and generously supporting various aspects of the author's scientific efforts in the plant tumor field over the past decade. I can only hope that the attempted synthesis that follows will, in small part at least, serve to justify the confidence that they have over the years placed in plant tumor research.

Acknowledgment is also made to *Science* for permission to use the illustration shown in Figure 1 of the article "Reversion in Hamster Cells Transformed by Rous Sarcoma Virus," by Ian Macpherson, *Science*, Vol. 148, pp. 1731–1733, 25 June 1965, Copyright 1965 by the American Association for the Advancement of Science; to Springer-Verlag, Vienna, for permission to use my illustrations previously published as Figures 2, 3, and 6 in "Morphology and Physiology of Plant Tumors," *Protoplasmatologia*, Vol. 10, Heft 5a, pp. 1–93, Springer, 1958; and to Basic Books, Inc., for permission to use my illustrations previously published as Figures 1 and 2 in "The Origin of the Plant Tumor Cell," in *Growth in Living Systems*, edited by M. X. Zarrow, © 1961 by Basic Books, Inc., Publishers, New York.

ARMIN C. BRAUN

The Rockefeller University
New York, New York
November 1968

CONTENTS

CHAPTER I

Introduction to the Tumor Problem

Introductory Remarks

It is likely that no biological problem has received more attention than that pertaining to cancer and other neoplastic diseases. A truly massive literature has accumulated, and a vast array of facts and observations relative to that subject has been recorded during the past century. Despite this enormous effort we find a certain pessimism expressed about progress that leads to an understanding of the basic cellular mechanism underlying the tumorous state. Peyton Rous, for example, commented in his Harvey Lecture that "the tumor problem is the last stronghold of metaphysics in medicine" where the mind can speculate almost at will formulating new hypotheses on causation (423). This evaluation of the problem was, of course, made before the advent of modern molecular biology with its revolutionary concepts and great promise. Yet, in 1966, Rubin (432) wrote:

Any serious attempt to evaluate the current state of our knowledge about cancer leads us to some rather dismal conclusions. One of the most depressing things about cancer research is that we have foisted the delusion upon ourselves and upon the public that there has indeed been rapid progress in this field. This delusion has been nurtured by the assumption that knowledge which has accumulated so rapidly in certain fields of biology . . . is somehow immediately and directly applicable to the cancer problem. Thus we have expropriated various bits of information from selected fields of biology, depending on which is the fashion of the day, and applied them with little or no modification to an explanation of how cells become malignant.

One might, I think, reasonably ask whether the evidence justifies such a cynical view of the progress that has been made in our understanding of the basic cellular mechanisms that underlie tumorigenesis.

Many would agree that it does. Yet an answer to that question would appear to depend largely on the level at which the problem is being analyzed. To a pathologist, for example, a demonstration that all tumors are caused by viruses might provide an intellectually satisfying answer. Yet such a finding, although doubtless of great practical value, would in itself tell us almost nothing about the cellular changes which are the immediate causes of malignant behavior. Similarly, a classical geneticist might be quite content with the knowledge that tumors generally are caused by gene mutations at the nuclear level. This knowledge again would offer no clue to what a mutation does in a cell to alter its behavior. It would appear necessary, therefore, to determine the nature of the heritable cellular changes at a physiological and biochemical level if an understanding of the basic mechanisms underlying the tumorous state is to be achieved.

One of the most puzzling aspects of the tumor problem is concerned with the multiplicity of diverse physical, chemical, and biological agencies that are capable of bringing about essentially the same end result. These agencies, with the possible exception of certain of the viruses, are concerned only with the inception of tumors and do not appear to be involved in the continued abnormal proliferation of the tumor cells once the conversion of normal cells to tumor cells has been accomplished. The implication of these findings appears to be that all the diverse agencies ultimately affect a common cellular mechanism(s) which, once deranged, urges the cells to continued abnormal proliferation. As Latarjet (300) points out, malignancy often expresses itself in ways which are independent of causative agents. From a clinical and pathological point of view nothing distinguishes the lymphomas produced in mice by X rays, carcinogenic chemicals, or viruses. There is, moreover, reason to believe that in all cases the disease is the same with the same heritable alteration at the cellular level. If true, this would suggest that the underlying heritable change found in the several diversely initiated tumors ultimately converges at the same point in the cell. Where, then, could this hypothetical point be?

One of the most striking characteristics of all higher organisms is the extraordinary way in which all of their functional parts fall into a coherent, flexible, but definitely limited pattern. This characteristic is so ubiquitous that it is likely for the most part to be passed over unnoticed. Sometimes, however, this harmony of structure and function is forcibly brought to our attention by its sudden failure. This is never more true than in the neoplastic diseases of animals and plants, for here the characteristic feature of the disease is a breakdown of the morphogenetic controls that govern so precisely the growth of all normal cells within an organism. The questions as to what governs the growth of all normal cells within an organism and what is entailed in overcoming those restraints under conditions of neoplasia are fundamental and constitute the ultimate basis of the tumor problem generally. It is with an attempt to find definitive answers to those questions that the present discussion is concerned. An attempt will be made here to show that the tumor problem is fundamentally a problem of anomalous differentiation and that the cellular factors that are concerned with the regulation of normal developmental processes are also basically involved in maintaining the neoplastic state. Before getting into a detailed documentation of the evidence that will be presented here, we might appropriately delve briefly into the history of the tumor problem and thus establish the fundamental concepts upon which modern cancer research is based.

The Development of Fundamental Concepts

Although as pointed out by Ewing (175), "The Ancients knew cancer well," modern research on the tumor problem may be considered to have been initiated by Johannes Müller in 1838 (367, 224). At about the time that the cell theory was first clearly formulated by Schleiden and Schwann, Müller demonstrated that tumors consisted of the abnormal growth of cells. His observation that cancer is cellular has remained to this day the basis of cancer research. From that time onward, the history of the tumor problem is a record of stages in the investigation of growth.

Virchow, a student of Müller, brilliantly carried forward the concept of cellular pathology which he founded on the doctrine *Omnis cellula e cellula* and defined more clearly some of the abnormalities which tumors reveal. He formulated the theory that chronic irritation was etiologically involved in the initiation of cancer (529). Waldeyer showed that metastatic tumors were the result of cell emboli and demonstrated the infiltration of cells of the primary tumor into blood and lymph vessels (537, 538). Ribbert advanced the hypothesis that cancers are due to the growth of small groups of epithelial cells which have been displaced by trauma or by growth abnormalities in the surrounding tissues (414). These cells, he believed, were not biologically different from normal cells but developed into tumors because of the unusual conditions into which they were placed. Ribbert insisted that no unusual powers of proliferation exist in cancer cells but that those cells, freed from the restraints of tissue tension, merely exhibit the powers of growth with which they are endowed from the ovum. Cohnheim's (124) theory of misplaced "embryonic rests," which for a time supplanted Virchow's irritation theory, was later largely abandoned as contrary to clinical observations.

In the last half of the nineteenth century numerous attempts were made to discover some parasite as the etiological agent in cancer. This work logically followed the success of bacteriologists in isolating causal organisms for many other diseases. Cancer was attributed at one time or another to almost every conceivable type of microbe but none of the alleged pathogens withstood critical investigation that is required to establish a causal relationship. By 1905, therefore, partly as a result of the failure of many attempts at isolation and partly because of the writings of Ribbert and others, the parasitic theory of cancer was discarded by almost all prominent workers in the field. It was during that period that Boveri (70, 71) presented the first evidence for his mutation theory of cancer—a theory that has many adherents to the present day.

Experimental studies that have proved to be important milestones in cancer research were those demonstrating the transplantability of the cancer cell. As early as 1889 both Hanau (227) and Wehr (543) successfully transplanted cancer cells, the former in rats and the latter in dogs. These studies were confirmed by Leo Loeb's work (317) on the rat thyroid sarcoma and, more particularly, by C. O. Jensen's brilliant investigations on the transplantability of mouse and, later, rat cancers (264, 265, 266). Some years later, in 1910, Jensen applied his talents to a study of the transplantability of certain plant tumors as well (267). From those studies he concluded that the formation of tumors in beets is based upon a continuous abnormal proliferative capacity of the cells. The effect of the tumor upon the growth of the beet, the abnormal chemical relationship of the tumor to the normal tissue, and the fact that the tumor studied was transplantable "remind one so much of the malignant tumors of animals, that a closer study of the biological relationships of these tumors would undoubtedly be profitable" (translated from the German) (267). Unfortunately, and largely because of the profound influence that Erwin F. Smith exerted in the field, the work of Jensen was widely ignored and was not again seriously considered until about thirty years later.

The demonstration of the transplantability of tumors gave impetus to the problem of autonomy of the cancer cell, and Hauser in 1903 was among the first to explain tumor growth on the assumption that a profound change had occurred in the cells that made up a malignant tumor (231). He regarded such tumors as being composed of a new race of cells and recognized their independence.

The Experimental Production of Cancer

Chemical, Physical, and Biological Agencies in the Initiation of Cancer

The great fundamental advance in twentieth-century cancer research was, however, the experimental production of cancer. Although, as indicated above, by the turn of the century the parasitic theory of cancer had been largely abandoned, there appeared shortly thereafter several contributions of far-reaching interest. One of these, although not dealing with animal cancer, was published in 1907 by Erwin F. Smith and C. O. Townsend (461). These workers found that a specific bacterium was responsible for the initiation of a rapidly developing neoplastic growth that is commonly known as the crown gall disease of plants. The isolation and characterization of a tumor-inducing bacterium shortly after the turn of the present century attracted considerable interest among pathologists generally because at the time of that discovery no animal tumor had as yet been produced experimentally. In 1913 Smith was awarded a certificate of honor by the American Medical Association for his work on cancer in plants. American pathologists further honored him in 1925 by electing him President of the American Association for Cancer Research.

For a period of about twenty years following his discovery, Smith made detailed comparative studies of crown gall and malignant animal tumors and found, as had Jensen, that these two types of growth had much in common. There appeared, however, to be one fundamental difference. Smith insisted, despite Jensen's beautiful studies of which he was fully aware, that the continued unregulated proliferation of the crown gall tumor cell was dependent upon continued stimulation by the inciting bacterium. By the middle 1920s, therefore, crown gall was not generally accepted by oncologists as being comparable to true animal tumors because, as described by Smith, this plant disease appeared to be simply a bacterial-stimulated hyperplasia and not a truly independent growth as are most animal cancers. It was not until 1942 that unequivocal evidence was presented for the truly autonomous nature of the crown gall tumor cell (85, 555).

In 1908, one year after the discovery by Smith and Townsend, Ellermann and Bang in Denmark demonstrated that cell-free filtrates of a chicken leukemia would transmit the disease (169). This important discovery attracted little attention among oncologists because at that time leukemias were not considered to be neoplastic diseases.

The papers published by Rous in 1910 (421, 422) dealing with fowl sarcomas which are transmissible by means of cell-free filtrates represent very fundamental discoveries. These findings are of particular significance because, as Andrewes (21) states, they render "untenable most of the arguments which had been built up to show that the parasitic theory of cancer *could* not be true." Although these solid neoplasms were at first considered by some not to be true tumors but rather virus-induced hyperplasias, they have in recent years gained considerable importance and at present the virus theory of the causation of cancer is one of the main concepts advanced in discussions on the etiology of the malignant state. Dr. Rous was honored some fifty years after his discovery by receiving the highest recognition that a scientist can attain.

Chronic irritation as a factor in the initiation of tumor growth has long been recognized. As early as 1775 Percivall Pott described scrotal cancer in chimney sweeps, due presumably to the continued contact of soot with the skin of the worker (400). Devergie, in 1857, described for the first time the relationship between skin cancer and lupus, a chronic tuberculous skin disease (150). With the development of the coal tar industry in the middle of the last century, an abundance of clinical evidence became available establishing certain products of the coal tar industry as causative agents in the genesis of cancer. Rehn in 1895 (410), among others, reported on the high incidence of cancer of the bladder among workers in the aniline dye industry. Maxwell in 1879 (344) described Kangri burn cancer and Wyss (574) called attention somewhat later to the induction of skin cancer by repeated X-ray burns. These clinical observations were supported by experimental evidence when in 1910 to 1912 Marie, Clunet, and Raulot-Lapointe (337, 338, 339) reported that they had produced experimentally a spindle-cell sarcoma of the rat by the application of heavy doses of X-irradiation. These authors described the dosage and intervals of treatment required to produce the malignant tumor.

In the now classical experiments of Yamagiwa and Ichikawa (576) cancer was first produced on the ears of rabbits by the application over long periods of time of gas-works tar. By painting the inner surface of rabbits' ears every second or third day for a period of about a year, these investigators obtained many papillomas and a few unquestionable carcinomas. This work together with an abundance of confirmatory evidence from many laboratories leaves little doubt that such tar products are instrumental in inducing the formation of tumors. These experiments were followed by the isolation of pure chemical compounds from the active tars which were capable of inducing malignant disease in experimental animals. Kennaway and Cook, together with their collaborators, were especially productive in this field (130, 238, 278, 279). In 1933 they isolated and identified 3,4-benzpyrene as a biologically active component of coal tar. From 1,2,5,6-dibenzanthracene, another substance isolated in 1930 from tar and which in itself is not very carcinogenic, a number of highly active derivatives were produced. Among the most powerful of these was methylcholanthrene, which bears a structural relationship to the sterols, bile acids, and sex hormones. This compound attracted particular interest because Wieland and Dane (556) and later Fieser and collaborators (180) showed that the bile acids can be transformed by chemical means into methylcholanthrene. It was thus proposed that cancer-producing hydrocarbons may arise in organisms by the abnormal metabolism of cholesterol and the bile acids.

This hypothesis was tested by Schabad (445, 446) who employed extracts of liver from cancer patients, since bile acids are synthesized in the liver. Such liver extracts were tested in mice and found to elicit a significant increase in the number of tumors found in various organs such as liver, kidney, lung, and mammary gland, as well as at the site of application. Some tumors were also produced in mice that were treated with similar preparations obtained from persons who did not have cancer. Later, Kleinenberg, Neufach, and Schabad (290) reported that extracts of lungs are at least as effective as those from liver. These studies leave little doubt that the human body contains and perhaps synthesizes carcinogenic substances. Because of the solubility properties of the compounds used by Schabad and others it is not unlikely that the carcinogen was cholesterol or one of its derivatives (384).

Numerous structurally different chemical compounds, in addition to the carcinogenic hydrocarbons, have been demonstrated to be tumorigenic over the years. Among these might be mentioned α- and β-naphthylamine and benzidine as well as aniline, which have been implicated in the production of bladder cancer in men working in the dye industry. The azo compounds, of which p-dimethylaminoazobenzene (butter yellow) and 4′amino-2,3′-azotoluene are representatives, are well-known liver tumor-inducing substances, especially in rats. Urethane, which is structurally another very different type of compound, increases significantly the number of lung adenomas in the mouse. The alkylating carcinogens NN-di(2-chloroethyl)methylamine and tri(2-chloroethyl)amine have been found to give rise to local sarcomas, adenocarcinomas of the lung, leukemias, angiosarcomas, and osteogenic sarcomas, while the cross-linking agents such as ethyleneimine and its numerous derivatives, as well as 2,4,6-triethyleneimino-1,3,5,triazine (TEM) and 1,4-dimethanesulphonyloxybutane (Myleran), are also carcinogenic in laboratory animals.

In addition to cholesterol and its derivatives, the estrogens represent potent endogenously produced carcinogens when administered to experimental animals. Other naturally occurring substances such as lard, olive oil, and arachis oil have been found to be weakly carcinogenic in certain test systems.

It has been discovered that plastics of various types including bakelite discs, cellophane, polyethylene, polyvinyl chloride, dacron, nylon, polystyrene, and commercial silicone films evoke sarcomas in rats when implanted in the tissues. The fact that not only these plastics but also stainless steel films are effective in eliciting tumors suggests that some physical condition rather than a chemical reaction is responsible for the sarcomatous change in these instances.

Among the inorganic substances shown to be carcinogenic are asbestos, arsenic, chromates, cobalt, beryllium, nickel carbonyl, and selenium. These are but a few of the almost endless catalogue of organic and inorganic substances found to be effective in eliciting tumors. They would appear to have little, if anything, in common from a structural or functional point of view and yet they accomplish essentially the same end result, i.e., the transformation of a normal cell into a tumor cell.

In addition to the chemical carcinogens such physical agents as ultraviolet rays, X rays, and radioactive substances (such as radium, plutonium, mesothorium and radiothorium, strontium 89, iodine 131), have been shown to be effective carcinogens (272).

Besides the chemical and physical agents, biological agents of the most diverse types have been implicated in tumor initiation. Mention has already been made of the specific bacterium, *Agrobacterium tumefaciens,* that initiates the non-self-limiting neoplastic disease of plants commonly known as the crown gall disease. This bacterium elaborates a tumor-inducing principle that regularly converts normal plant cells into tumor cells in short periods of time. Once the cellular transformation has been accomplished, the continued abnormal and autonomous proliferation of the host cells becomes an automatic process that is entirely independent of any recognizable infectious agent. It is, in fact, possible to kill selectively, by means of a thermal treatment, the inciting bacterium before there is the slightest evidence of tumefaction at the point of inoculation and yet if the bacteria are allowed to act at a wound site for as little as three to four days before being destroyed thermally, rapidly growing fully autonomous and transplantable tumors will regularly develop (74, 75). This type of study provides unequivocal evidence that a factor of very considerable biological interest passes from the bacteria to the host cells and brings about a profound and heritable change in the subsequent behavior of the affected cells.

In the animal field, among the earliest parasites to be implicated in the initiation of cancer was *Schistosoma haematobium,* the causal agent of schistosomiasis. The eggs of this parasite are deposited in the veins of the bladder and occasionally in the rectum. They give rise to a cystitis with hematuria, anemia, and, in chronic cases, calculus formation and the development of papillomas which may become malignant. Unquestionable cases of this type were described by Virchow as early as 1888 (530) and it has been estimated that cancer results in about 5% of all persons afflicted with genitourinary schistosomiasis, a very significant number in view of the frequency of this disease in certain parts of the world where it is endemic. Askanazy in 1900 (22) described cases of cancer of the liver of man resulting as a consequence of infestation with another parasite, *Opisthorchis felineus,* a liver fluke. This work was not, however, put on a firm experimental basis until 1913 when Johannes Fibiger announced that he was able to produce true cancers in the stomach of rats by feeding them nematodes found in muscles of certain species of cockroaches (179). Metastases were observed by Fibiger in distant organs in which no nematodes or eggs were found. In these studies, then, carcinomas which gave rise to metastases were produced experimentally. Since the publication of this work the subject of "worm cancers" has been investigated not only by Fibiger but also by many others in a variety of different systems (384).

The mechanism by which these parasites incite neoplastic growth is not known. Fibiger believed, however, that the carcinoma with which he worked was initiated by the irritating action of some chemical substance elaborated by the nematode. Similar arguments have been raised in the case of a rat liver sarcoma, which is caused by a tapeworm of the cat, since the tumor in this instance does not appear unless the worm remains alive in the liver cysts for a period of about one year. Borrel (66), on the other hand, interpreted the results of Fibiger, his own, and those of others differently. He believed, without any real evidence, that there was a distinct cancer virus or viruses and that the parasites were merely the carrier of such agents. Borrel was apparently a man of uncanny perception. Oberling (384) states:

Yet Borrel made predictions that should have struck, as they did me, all those who were privileged to discuss with him the problems of cancer. He foresaw that there would be failures at times in attempts to produce malignant growths with *Spiroptera,* insisted that parasites take part in the spreading of viruses, and suspected from the first that in the so-called hereditary cancer of mice something other than genetic factors may be transmitted. More than once I have heard him suggest the passage of some agent by way of the milk.

These predictions, which have now all been realized, were made at a time when it required the greatest courage to maintain the virus hypothesis of the causation of cancer.

This, then, brings us again to by far the most important class of oncogenic agents of biological nature, the viruses. Although, as indicated earlier, a number of chicken viruses had been shown to be etiologically involved in leukemia and solid tumor production shortly after the turn of the present century, this field did not again receive much attention until the 1930s. It was not until 1932 that the known number and host range of oncogenic viruses began to expand. In that year Richard Shope found small nodules which proved to be fibromas under the skin of the front and hind paws of a wild cottontail rabbit shot near Princeton, N. J. (451). He was able to transmit these tumors by means of cell-free extracts to cottontail and domestic rabbits. In 1933 Shope described another mammalian tumor of viral origin (452); this virus causes benign, epidermal papillomas in the common wild cottontail rabbits in the southwestern part of the United States. Very occasionally these benign growths become malignant in their natural hosts. This happened much more frequently when papillomas were initiated in domestic rabbits by the Shope virus. While the papillomas are very similar in morphology, the derivative carcinomas varied widely.

Seven of these malignant derivatives, which are now called the VX carcinomas, have been transplanted serially for many years and strenuous efforts have been made to isolate a "cancer virus" from them, without success. This failure is the more impressive because six of the seven cancers have consistently yielded the papilloma virus. The seventh, the VX2 carcinoma, which has now been serially transplanted for more than 30 years, contained an antigen of the papilloma virus throughout its first 3.5 years of maintenance, its rabbit hosts being completely resistant to reinoculation with the virus. On the other hand, after 4.5 years not even this evidence of the presence of the virus was left and the animals carrying the tumors have regularly proved to be as susceptible to reinoculation with it as are normal animals. These findings indicate, then, that the Shope papilloma virus acts only to initiate the production of papillomas and that the secondarily derived carcinomas presumably arise from other causes.

In 1934 Lucké (323) described renal adenocarcinomas to be of unusually common occurrence in leopard frogs found in the New England States and he and others described the virus responsible for this notably malignant disease. Lucké was able to transmit this disease by inoculating tumor tissue that had been desiccated or stored in 50% glycerine for three weeks. The resulting tumors occurred in the kidneys and not at the injection site. From these studies Lucké concluded that the cause of this malignancy was a virus (324). It was not, however, until 1956 that Duryee (163), and in 1964 Lunger (325), presented more conclusive evidence for the viral etiology of this tumor. The frog virus acts only on the convoluted tubules of the kidney, producing carcinoma of a distinctive kind. Often the malignant cells contain acidophilic intranuclear inclusion bodies, but nearly as often these are lacking and the growths then resemble classical cancers.

A most interesting virus, the Bittner milk factor or, as it is sometimes called, mouse mammary tumor virus, was first clearly recognized in 1936 (53) although earlier studies had suggested the involvement of some extrachromosomal factor in the etiology of the disease. For many years, pure highly inbred strains of mice had been developed with a very high mammary tumor incidence which was independent of known external factors and thus appeared to be a genetic characteristic of the mouse strain. However, when high- and low-incidence mammary tumor strains were bred, it was found that F_1 females foster-nursed on mothers from the high-incidence mammary tumor strain developed many mammary tumors. On the other hand, those foster-nursed on mothers from the low-incidence strain developed very few mammary tumors. These studies indicated, therefore, that there was some extrachromosomal factor that was transmitted from mother to daughter in the strains of mice with a high incidence of mammary tumors. Such a factor could have been transmitted through the placenta, in the cytoplasm of the ovum, or after birth through the milk. Bittner found that the causative agent was transmitted through the milk (54, 55). The agent was later found to pass through bacteria-proof filters and could, therefore, reasonably be considered to be a virus (56). Mammary cancer in mice was, therefore, a communicable disease.

The mammary tumor virus was found, however, to be only one of several essential factors in a very complex etiology. The virus appears to do no more than to cause tiny growths, known as "hyperplastic nodules," in the mammary glands of susceptible females. These nodules are conditional adenomas, dependent for their growth on hormonal influences. However, carcinomas are very often derived from the nodules. In this way they become responsible for the frequency of mammary cancers in mice carrying the milk virus. The more effective the virus is in causing adenomas, the more frequently do malignant growths arise from them. Thus, we see that the development of breast carcinomas in mice is probably due to the influence of three factors: (1) an inherited breast cancer susceptibility, (2) the Bittner milk virus, and (3) a hormonal influence.

Here, as in the case of the Shope papilloma, no "cancer virus" has been isolated from the carcinomas that developed from the adenomas. The malignant derivatives have never yielded anything except the milk virus, which may be carried along in the tissues throughout years of serial transplantation, only to be lost eventually. Thus, the milk virus is like the papilloma virus in that it initiates only benign tumors from which the cancers arise.

In 1944 the first non-self-limiting neoplastic disease of viral origin in plants was described by Lindsay Black (57). The virus of this disease, now known as the wound tumor disease, is transmitted in nature by agallian leafhoppers of several species. It can also be transmitted mechanically if a high enough concentration of virus is present in the inoculum. The virus replicates in both its animal and plant hosts. A survey of potential plant hosts has indicated that at least 43 species in 20 families support growth of the virus. Of these, however, only three develop tumorous overgrowths. In *Portulaca oleracea* L. the tops of infected plants bear no symptoms while numerous small tumors are formed on the roots. Sorrel (*Rumex acetosa* L.) and sweet clover (*Melilotus alba* Desr.) produce large tumors which show a capacity for unlimited disorganized growth both *in situ* and *in vitro*. Investigations on sweet clover demonstrated that the heredity of the host plant affects the number, size, distribution, and morphology of the tumors (58). In some strains root tumors may be so numerous and large that they fuse together, while in other strains they may be so small and inconspicuous as to be easily overlooked. Stem reaction in some clones involves the formation of many large tumors; in other clones stem tumors rarely appear. Hereditary influences on stem and root may act independently. For example, one clone produces large tumors on stems and roots while another produces many large root tumors but only a few stem tumors.

That the genetic basis which causes a clone to be highly predisposed to tumor formation involves not merely a susceptibility to the virus but also a tendency toward tumorous proliferation is indicated by the inbred B21 line of sweet clover. This line, which appears to be inclined to tumor formation, produced five spontaneous tumors over a period of time (313). That these did not represent accidental infections was demonstrated by the facts that no root tumors were observed on plants which ordinarily would have a profusion of root tumors if infected, and that these plants showed no immunity to infection by the wound tumor virus. The five spontaneous tumors had, moreover, a similar and distinct histology which was different from that characteristic of virus-induced tumors. The authors compare sweet clover line B21 with strain C3Hb of mice which have lost the mammary carcinoma virus and yet show an inherent tendency to develop mammary carcinomas (237).

In addition to the virus and the hereditary constitution of the host, the expression of the tumorous aspect of the disease is limited to areas of irritation such as those resulting from a wound, increased hormone levels, etc. Thus, although a plant may be systemically infected by the virus, tumors arise only at sites of active cell division such as those resulting from irritation accompanying a wound. It has been found, moreover, that the tumor tissue of sweet clover contains about one hundred times more virus than does normal tissue. This subject has been reviewed in detail by Black (60). Certain aspects of this disease will be considered in greater detail in Chapter IV.

By the early 1950s evidence had thus begun to accumulate indicating that tumors in many different organisms are caused by viruses. This naturally raised the larger question of whether the generality of tumors are due to viruses, a belief voiced most strongly by Oberling (384). Yet all of the oncogenic animal viruses known up to that time were narrowly limited in cell types which they transformed and were effective in only one or, at most, a few closely related species. With such specificity it would have been necessary to postulate a myriad of such agents to account for the multiplicity of different tumors observed in even a single animal species such as man. It was at that time, however, that a number of discoveries were made which provided the key to the enormous progress that has been made in virus tumor research during the past decade.

In 1951 Gross reported the production of leukemia in C3H mice inoculated soon after birth with cell-free extracts of leukemic tissues from AK mice (216). Although at first these observations were confirmed with some difficulty, a number of distinct strains of mouse leukemia virus have now been identified. Some of these produce lymphatic leukemia, others myeloid leukemia, while a third group causes a disease which is not easy to classify but appears to be a reticulum cell plus erythroblastic leukemia.

During the course of their studies on mouse leukemia Gross (217) and Stewart (484) independently observed that suckling mice inoculated with cell-free extract of leukemic tissue from AK strain mice developed parotid tumors. It was soon found that these leukemic extracts contained two viruses, one of which produced leukemia when injected into very young mice while the other, which became known as the polyoma virus, produced solid tumors when similarly injected. The polyoma virus was soon recognized as being very different from the tumor viruses discovered earlier. In contrast to the previously isolated viruses, which appeared to be more or less species-specific and to produce only one type of tumor, the polyoma virus initiated a great variety of tumors in many different species. In one group of 117 mice inoculated soon after birth with the polyoma virus, 23 different and distinct types of tumors were found (485). As well as in mice, this virus initiates tumors, under appropriate conditions following inoculation, in both Chinese and Syrian hamsters, rabbits, rats, ferrets, guinea pigs, and *Rattus* (*Mastomys*) *natalensis,* the multimammate mouse. These findings exerted an enormous impact on virus tumor research. Peyton Rous commented on them by stating: "Nature, as is her way, has hit us a wallop just when we least expected it. Now at last we can think, but as yet only think, in terms of a relatively few viruses, each of wide scope, as possibly causing the generality of tumors" (424).

The polyoma virus, unlike the earlier studied tumor viruses, appeared to have many characteristics in common with those viruses which produce nontumorous diseases or are orphan viruses. Since tissue cultures of monkey kidney cells, which are commonly used in

↑ preparing virus vaccines such as the polio vaccine, were known to contain a number of orphan viruses as contaminants, Eddy and her colleagues considered the possibility that one or more of those contaminating viruses might be of a tumor-producing type (166, 167). These workers prepared extracts from pooled rhesus monkey kidney cells and inoculated them into newborn hamsters. After a period of 118 days undifferentiated sarcomas appeared not only at the injection site but also in the lungs and kidneys of certain of the animals. The tumor virus proved to be identical with simian virus 40 (SV40) (202) that had been observed by Sweet and Hilleman in 1960 (502). Hamsters and the multimammate mouse are the only species known in which the SV40 virus has been shown to induce tumors. Man is, however, susceptible to non-neoplastic infection by this virus and was frequently infected by contaminated virus vaccines prepared from monkey kidney tissue cultures before this danger was recognized. Cells of human patients with Fanconia's anemia are also readily transformed by SV40 in tissue culture (518).

It has recently been shown that at least eight types of the commonly found human adenovirus can induce tumors in certain animals such as newborn hamsters, rats, certain strains of mice, and *Mastomys*. The first of these, type 12, was found to produce sarcomas at the injection site in newborn hamsters after a latent period of one to three months (523). It was subsequently found by others that types 7, 18, and 31 were also quite effective in eliciting tumors. Although infective virus is not found in adenovirus-induced tumors, the cells contain a specific complement-fixing antigen (253).

The thoughts recorded here on the tumor viruses are in part those expressed by K. E. K. Rowson in Chapter 7 of *The Biology of Cancer* (E. J. Ambrose and F. J. C. Roe, eds.), p. 124, Van Nostrand, London and Princeton, 1966. Viral-host cell interactions will be considered in Chapter IV.

The Synergistic Effect of Biological, Chemical, and Physical Oncogens. The fact that chemical carcinogens can enhance the effect of a virus has long been known from the studies of Rous and Friedewald (427). These investigators showed that the application of chemical carcinogens to rabbits carrying the Shope papilloma virus resulted in the rapid production of cancers and these were always of the same type that would have appeared at a much later date as a result of virus action alone. Similarly, Duran-Reynals found that when chickens affected with an ordinary virus, in this case the fowl pox virus, were treated with methylcholanthrene, skin neoplasms resulted. These new growths appeared at a time when the carcinogen alone would have caused nothing. Thus, the neoplastic growths seemed to have resulted from an interaction between the fowl pox virus and the carcinogen (162). Recently, several human viruses, notably that of herpes simplex, which are ordinarily non-neoplastic have been found to induce tumors in mice previously painted with chemical carcinogens in an amount too small to be oncogenic in themselves (343, 504).

Another type of interaction between chemical and physical oncogens and the viruses raises the interesting possibility that agents of the former type may activate latent viruses within cells. Gross (218) and Lieberman and Kaplan (307) have reported that following small doses of X-radiation to certain mice, leukemia viruses could be demonstrated which could not be demonstrated in animals prior to irradiation. These results suggest, then, that certain mice carry a latent virus which can be activated by small doses of X-radiation. Similarly, McIntosh and Selbie (351) and Oberling and Guérin (385) have claimed to have obtained active filtrates from fowl sarcomas induced in the first instance with tar and in the second with methylcholanthrene. Such sporadic findings, which attest to an interaction of carcinogens and viruses, are as yet far too limited and thus cannot be considered more than suggestive in support of the hypothesis that chemical and physical carcinogens may exert their effects by rendering, either directly or indirectly, latent viruses actively neoplastic and in this way account for the initiation of the generality of tumors.

In addition to the physical, chemical, and biological agencies described above, cancer cells sometimes arise as a result of growing normal cells for prolonged periods of time in culture. The actual demonstration of the neoplastic transformation in isolated systems stems from the pioneering studies of Gey (200, 201) and Earle and collaborators (164, 372, 442). These studies doubtless represent a milestone in cancer research and their significance has been heightened by the quite unexpected finding that no known carcinogen needs to be added to the culture medium in order to achieve the neoplastic transformation. A similar phenomenon, known as habituation, has been reported in the plant field (195, 310).

[Thus we are confronted with a most perplexing situation. The transformation of a normal cell into a tumor cell may occur in culture without the influence of any recognizable carcinogen; it may be accomplished by physical agents, by very simple inorganic or organic substances, by more complex organic molecules, and by highly complex biological agencies such as the viruses. Is there, then, a common denominator that can account for these unusual observations? The answer is probably Yes, and if that is true, it must be looked for in the altered metabolism of the transformed cell and, more particularly, in that area of metabolism concerned with the regulation of cell growth and division.]

Hereditary Factors in Cancer

In addition to the multiplicity of proximate causes described above, the genetic constitution of a host appears to be of central importance in determining whether or not a tumor will be produced. The intervention of hereditary factors in the genesis of many tumors has now been demonstrated beyond any reasonable question of doubt. This is evidenced most clearly in the high- and low-incidence cancer lines of inbred strains of certain mice where in the high-incidence lines virtually every member will die of cancer at a predestined time, and even the very site of the origin of the new growth is commonly predetermined. Inbreeding, of course, provides "biological magnification" and leads to higher genetic resolution. Close inbreeding has now been carried to such an extreme that certain investigators (109) have, in fact, argued that the highly inbred mouse is a wholly artificial creature, a man-made artifact and, hence, has little to do with reality. Yet the cancer problem is so elusive that every clue must be followed and much of significance has been learned with the use of the inbred strains of mice.

The pioneer work of Maud Slye (460) as well as that of Clara Lynch (326) and Marsh (342), and extended later by the studies of Little (316), Strong (497), Woolley (573), and Heston (236), have demonstrated the existence in inbred mice of large numbers of genes determining or affecting cancer-proneness for many types of tumors.

The conclusions to be drawn from the genetic studies on mice are at one and the same time simple and sweeping. It has been found that all types of mouse cancer thus far investigated by appropriate and adequate techniques have some genetic basis. It must be recognized, however, that cancer-proneness, like other characters, is affected by environmental influences. Thus, in mice a restricted diet reduces the incidence of most tumors, notably mammary cancer. Riboflavin, on the other hand, reduces the incidence of azo-dye-induced hepatomas in rats, while a low cystine diet reduces the incidence of methylcholanthrene-induced leukemia in mice. Needless to say, many other examples of this type could be cited.

Although man cannot be subjected to experimental breeding, there is every reason to believe that there is a strong heritable factor determining cancer-proneness in man as well as in the mouse. This is perhaps most clearly shown in comparative studies of identical and fraternal twins. Identical (homologous) twins, since presumably they come from the same fertilized ovum, are two individuals endowed with identical heredity. Fraternal twins, on the other hand, are merely two individuals born at the same time of the same parents and thus are no more similar in their hereditary make-up than ordinary brothers and sisters would be.

McFarland and Meade collected twenty reports of tumors occurring in identical twins (350). In every case reported the tumor was present in each twin of the pair and it was, moreover, of the same type occurring in the same organ. Further, the tumor was found to occur at approximately the same age and no instance was found in this study of one twin having a tumor without the other having the same type of tumor. The twins were usually not living together and were often many miles apart and thus not subject to the same environmental conditions. Are these findings more than coincidence? McFarland and Meade, themselves, point to the famous twins who each lost a left leg during battle in the American Civil War. Yet, when one considers not only the data of McFarland and Meade but also that of Busk, Clemmesen, and Nielsen (110) and Darlington and Mather (140a), there can be little doubt that cancers in identical twins are generally of the same type, at the same site, and frequently occur at the same age. Certain types of tumors such as mammary and uterine cancer show no difference in concordance between identical and fraternal twins, thus suggesting that genetic predisposition to them is negligible. Incidence of gastric cancer, on the other hand, shows evidence of a marked genetic predisposition.

Through an analysis of human pedigrees, medical genetics has also demonstrated certain types of tumors that are determined genetically by single alleles. These include, among others, xeroderma pigmentosum which has been found to result from a recessive and partially sex-linked gene. The skin of persons homozygous for this recessive gene invariably develops malignant tumors but only if exposed to strong sunlight. What is obviously transmitted in this instance is not the cancer but the gene which then predisposes the skin exposed to sunlight to the development of cancer. Other examples of this type are the semidominant (with effects in the hemizygous state) retino-blastoma as well as multiple intestinal polyposis which almost invariably develop into cancers. Many other examples of hereditary predisposition to tumor formation are found in Ford (185), Gorer (209), Kemp (276), Lynch (327), Snyder (464), and Woolley (573).

Tumors Due to Genetic Imbalance of Wide Crosses. Crosses between different related species of animals and plants often result in genetic imbalances in which growth abnormalities of various kinds may be found. It is not surprising, therefore, that in certain hybrids genetic tumors regularly occur because of an upset of the balance between growth and the regulation of growth. Tumors that develop as a result of hybridization may be considered to support the so-called imbalance theory of cancer, which holds that all organisms need to evolve systems of growth regulation and that tumors arise when imbalance in favor of growth passes a certain threshold. Thus, genetic imbalance is expressed in developmental imbalance.

Among the most thoroughly analyzed cases of this type are the so-called Kostoff genetic tumors that develop spontaneously in certain interspecific hybrids within the genus *Nicotiana*. This subject has recently been reviewed by Ahuja (7). When, for example, two non-tumor-forming species such as *Nicotiana glauca* and *Nicotiana langsdorffii* are crossed and the seed of the hybrid sown, the resulting plants commonly develop normally during the period of their active growth and in the absence of irritation. Once these hybrids reach maturity and terminal growth ceases, a profusion of tumors invariably develops from all parts of the plant. These tumors commonly arise at points of natural irritation. Feeding the plants radioactive phosphorus or irradiating them hastens the onset of tumors and increases significantly the number of tumors that develops (472, 473). Chemical irritation may also initiate tumors. Kehr and Smith report that leaves accidentally splashed with a mixture of turpentine, whiting, and white lead developed tumors at almost every spot where droplets of the spray mixture had struck the leaf (275).

All attempts to isolate a causative agent such as a bacterium, a virus, or a fungus have failed. This evidence indicates that this pathological condition is genetically inherent in the hybrid plant and requires only some nonspecific stimulus, which does not affect the parent species in the same way, to elicit tumor formation. More than forty tumor-producing hybrid combinations have thus far been described within the genus *Nicotiana* (368). It has been found, moreover, that parents of the tumorous hybrids can be divided into two groups which have been arbitrarily designated as the "plus" and "minus" groups. If an intragroup cross is made between two "plus" species or between two "minus" species, the resulting offspring will not develop tumors. On the other hand, crosses between a "plus" species and a "minus" species produce tumor-bearing offspring. Of a total of more than fifty such crosses studied, very few exceptions to this rule have been found. From these studies it was concluded that the critical contributions of the "plus" parents must differ from those of the "minus" parents. These contributions, although genetic in nature, must be reflected in parental metabolism.

An attempt to analyze the genetic basis of these tumors was made. Reciprocal crosses gave identical results, indicating that maternal cytoplasmic factors were not involved. Kehr and Smith (275, 274) bred a considerable number of diploid and polyploid combinations of *Nicotiana glauca* × *N. langsdorffii* and concluded from those studies that the tumor-forming nature of the hybrid remains relatively unchanged regardless of the ratio of *N. glauca* and *N. langsdorffii* chromosomes as long as one complete genome of each species is present in the hybrid. It was also found in those studies that no tumors developed when only one or a few of the twelve *glauca* chromosomes were present in addition to the diploid complement of *langsdorffii* chromosomes.

A quite similar situation, originally described by Häussler in 1928, is found in fish (232). In this instance the F_1 hybrids of certain species of the subgenera *Platypoecilus* (platyfish) and *Xiphophorus* (swordtail) regularly develop melanomas which may expand rapidly and may be fatal. In over twenty thousand specimens examined of either species no melanomas were found. The tumors in the hybrid arise from the large macromelanophores. Melanomas may develop in almost any part of the body. Extensive genetic studies have been carried out in this system. A study of those data reveals a significant relationship between the spatial association of genes and the effects they produce. The linkage of genes *RtSb* in the platyfish interacting with the *A* and *B* modifying genes of the swordtail determines the development of melanomas in their hybrids. Anders has postulated that the formation of melanomas in platyfish-swordtail hybrids results from a partial or total derepression and increased induction of a gene(s) (20).

An interesting mammalian case of this type was reported by Little in the cross between the wild mouse *Mus bacterianus* and an inbred strain of the domestic mouse *Mus musculus* (315). Here the incidence of multiple tumors in the F_1 hybrid was tenfold higher than the sum of the parents' incidences. Since these hybrids were sterile, no further genetic analyses could be made.

Other Concepts that Have Contributed to an Understanding of the Tumor Problem

Biological Concepts

Tumorigenesis as a Multi-step Process. The significant concept that carcinogenesis may under certain conditions be a discontinuous process consisting of several stages each with different characteristics had its origin in the studies of two independent groups of investigators. In 1941 Berenblum reported that chemical carcinogenesis in the mouse skin involves a two-step process (48). This investigator painted the skin of mice with a threshold dose of benzpyrene which in itself did not result in the development of tumors but which appeared to initiate sudden and apparently persistent changes in some of the mouse skin cells. These latent tumor cells could be made to develop into benign tumors by repeatedly applying a promoting agent or cocarcinogen such as croton oil. Malignancy appears to develop later and involves one or more additional steps.

In 1941 Rous and his associates (428, 329) also published papers on the induction of tumors in the skin of rabbits' ears with the use of either tar, benzpyrene or methylcholanthrene. The key experiments for Rous's theory of carcinogenesis as a two-step process, which he referred to as initiation and promotion, consisted in demonstrating that when rabbits' ears are tarred intermittently, the tumors which disappear after tarring is suspended may reappear at the same site when tarring is resumed. It was found, further, that when the tumors resulting from tarring regressed, they could be made to develop again, sometimes at precisely the same place, with noncarcinogenic stimuli such as wound healing or the application of chloroform or turpentine.

The results of both of these studies demonstrate, then, that a limited application of a chemical carcinogen used as an initiating agent will not alone result in the formation of tumors, or will result in benign growths that often regress. The chemical carcinogen, nevertheless, induces changes in the affected cells which when exposed repeatedly to irritants such as croton oil, chloroform, and turpentine or even to a wound healing response give rise to tumors that may eventually become malignant. Boutwell (67) has recently discussed this problem in detail and has concluded that (1) it is possible to breed mice selectively for susceptibility and resistance to initiation and promotion, (2) there are qualitative differences between the initiation and promotion processes, and (3) the formation process of benign and malignant tumors is divisible into three distinct operational steps. Evidence in support of a two-phase concept involving tumor inception and development was presented for the crown gall disease of plants in 1942 (82).

The study of neoplasia as a developmental process received its first clear experimental expression in papers published by Rous and Beard in 1935 (426) and by Greene several years later (212). The former described the progression of the virus-induced benign Shope papillomas into carcinomas, while Greene studied progressive steps leading to greater malignancy in certain transplantable tumors of the rabbit. Still later, Foulds (187) described the "growth and progression" of spontaneous mammary tumors in mice and proposed six general principles underlying tumor progression. These were listed as follows:

1. The independent progression of tumors. Different tumors in the same animal progress independently.
2. The independent progression of characters. Progression occurs independently in different characters in the same tumor.
3. Progression is independent of growth. Progression occurs in latent tumor cells and in tumors whose growth is arrested.

    Foulds has listed two notable corollaries of this third principle:

    (a) At its first clinical manifestation a tumor may be at any stage of progression.

    (b) Progression is independent of the size or clinical duration of a tumor.

4. Progression is continuous or discontinuous, by gradual change or by abrupt steps.
5. Progression follows one of alternative paths of development.
6. Progression does not always reach an endpoint within the lifetime of the host.

According to Foulds the most illuminating of these principles are those embodied in Rules 1, 2, and 5 which probably have a common basis revealed most clearly in Rule 2.

Tumor progression has also been found to occur in the crown gall disease of plants. In this instance various stages in the progression of the tumor can be obtained at will and the cellular changes underlying several of those stages have been defined experimentally. This matter will be considered in detail in Chapter III.

Biochemical Concepts

The three main biochemical concepts that have been proposed over the years to attempt to explain the basic mechanisms underlying tumorigenesis are the Warburg Hypothesis, the Greenstein Hypothesis, and the several versions of the Deletion Hypothesis postulated by members of the McArdle Memorial Laboratory at the University of Wisconsin (403, 403a).

The Warburg Hypothesis, which was first formulated in 1923 and which held the center of the stage for several decades, was based on the assumption that a universal correlation existed between aerobic glycolysis and the cancerous state (540). Warburg believes that cancer originates when a non-neoplastic cell develops an anaerobic metabolism as a means of survival after injury to its respiratory system. The data in support of this conclusion were provided in terms of the continued accumulation of lactic acid in the presence of oxygen and by the ability of cancer cells to incorporate amino acids under anaerobic conditions. Many angry words have been exchanged concerning the validity of the Warburg generalizations, with Weinhouse the chief antagonist (544). Serious questions concerning the universal correlation believed to exist between cancer and aerobic glycolysis were raised with the discovery of the so-called minimal deviation hepatomas (403a). These tumors represent the earliest stages of cancer cells in a transplantable and malignant form that have yet been found and for which the cell of origin is known. The results of studies on the glycolytic capacity of these tumors have clearly established that they do not remotely resemble the tumor tissues studied by Warburg. With respect to glycolysis the hepatomas studied (8, 9) resembled normal liver as closely as one sample of liver resembles another (403a). It is thus apparent that the Warburg generalization that a respiratory defect leading to aerobic glycolysis is the first and most important biochemical lesion in carcinogenesis is now open to very serious question.

The Greenstein Hypothesis (213), which many workers now feel has outlived its usefulness, states most simply that in tumors there is a general convergence of enzyme patterns leading to the biochemical uniformity of all tumor tissues. Nevertheless, the interesting new element introduced by Greenstein was the demonstration that each normal tissue had a characteristic pattern of enzymes if by pattern is meant the relative amounts of a series of qualitatively distinct enzyme functions. This finding was in contrast to the rather uniform pattern or relative amount of the same series of enzymes in a group of well-known transplantable tumor strains. It has, however, since been found that in transplantable tumors, as in normal tissue, there is a great diversity among the enzyme patterns (403a).

The Deletion Hypothesis in its various forms will be considered in some detail in Chapter IV. It might simply be stated here that the results thus far obtained with methods of cell hybridization have raised some very serious questions as to the usefulness of the deletion concepts as they relate to an understanding of the basic mechanisms underlying tumorigenesis generally.

Biochemists have in the past commonly assumed that any enzymatic or other biochemical changes that could be demonstrated in tumor cells were of immediate relevance to the carcinogenic change and often no attempt was made even to suggest how such observed differences might be related to the property of malignancy (403).

Distinguishing Characteristics of Neoplastic Cells

Malignancy is essentially a clinical concept and is used to describe the lethal behavior of certain tumors. Many independently variable characters enter into the expression of this complex phenomenon and these characters are subject to wide variations that require separate specification and study. This "dissociation of characters," as Hamperl (226) has called it, is exemplified by the "locally malignant" tumors that invade vigorously but rarely metastasize, by the metastasizing "benign" tumors that become widely distributed in a host despite a minimum of local invasions, and by certain benign tumors that are transplantable but that do not commonly invade or metastasize but rather continue to grow to huge size and ultimately cause death simply by overwhelming the host (see Fig. 1). It is thus possible with the three models described above to dissociate the capacity to invade, to metastasize, and simply to grow autonomously without either invading or metastasizing (187).

Among the more important characters commonly used to define malignancy are autonomy leading to unrestrained growth, transplant-ability, invasiveness, and metastasis. It is clear, however, that some of these characters such as invasiveness and the ability to metastasize may be acquired, sometimes relatively late, and can, therefore, be dismissed in a search for the earliest steps in carcinogenesis. This, then, leaves two characters, autonomy and transplantability, to be accounted for. Since transplantability is, in part at least, a reflection of the degree of autonomy that a cell has achieved, the cardinal feature underlying neoplastic growth generally would appear to be the acquisition by a cell of a capacity for autonomous growth. By autonomy is meant that a tumor cell determines its own activities

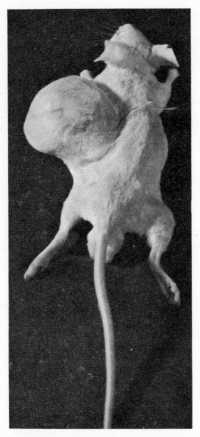

Fig. 1. Transplantable tumor (keratoma) of the type that does not invade neighboring tissues and does not metastasize but simply overwhelms and ultimately kills its host as a result of continued growth. The capacities of a tumor to invade and metastasize appear, therefore, to be secondarily acquired characteristics. (Courtesy of Dr. James S. Henderson.)

largely irrespective of the laws that govern so precisely the growth of all normal cells within an organism.

The property of autonomy may be expressed by both benign and malignant tumors. It has, in fact, been argued that the fundamental cellular processes underlying tumor growth may be revealed most clearly in benign tumors which represent neoplasia in its simplest and most uncomplicated form. Autonomy is not, however, a fixed and unvarying character but has many gradations ranging from very slow to very rapidly growing cell types. It is true, moreover, that many

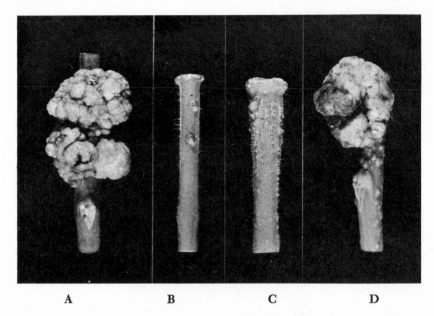

A   **B**   **C**   **D**

Fig. 2. An example of a hormone-dependent tumor in plants. **A.** Autonomous crown gall tumor. **B.** Hormone-dependent crown gall tumor. **C.** Response of control plant when hormone was applied to cut stem end. **D.** Response of hormone-dependent tumor when hormone was similarly applied to cut stem end of the plant. The hormone-dependent tumor continued to grow only as long as an exogenous source of the hormone was present.

types of normal cells grow at far faster rates than do most tumor cells. Normal regenerating liver cells, for example, grow much more rapidly than do hepatoma cells as evidenced by their more rapid uptake of radioactive phosphorus (97). Similarly, a squamous cell carcinoma of the skin or even a lymphoma after perhaps years of growth will rarely equal the size of a human fetus at term. It is thus not rate of growth but the development of a capacity for essentially unrestrained or autonomous growth that is important.

It is true, furthermore, that how a tumor develops in a host may be determined by the environment in which the tumor is growing. This is particularly well illustrated in the case of the so-called conditional or hormone-dependent tumors of plants (see Fig. 2), animals, and man. Conditional prostate or breast tumors, which may be highly malignant, grow only as long as the appropriate hormonal stimulus is present. When the specific stimulus is withdrawn growth stops and they regress, but when the stimulus is restored tumors will reoccur in the same place and with the same characters that they originally showed. Many conditional tumors undergo progression to a hormone-independent state if allowed sufficient time and thus they become true tumors. It can, therefore, be argued that any true tumor is merely a conditional tumor in which all of the conditions necessary for autonomous growth have been completely satisfied. This concept can, moreover, be considered independently of the malignancy of a tumor since, no matter how malignant the form of a tumor, if conditions necessary for its autonomous growth are withdrawn, it will regress.

Another distinguishing trait of malignant cells is the lack of perfect form and function exhibited by such cell types when compared with their normal counterparts. This characteristic is known as anaplasia which, as a descriptive term, is at home largely in the minds and literature of the classical pathologist. This loss of cellular characters, known as dedifferentiation, is sometimes erroneously referred to as a reversion of neoplastic cells to the embryonic state. While embryonic cells, even in their most undifferentiated form, respond exquisitely to controls provided by the organism and by one another, dedifferentiated cancer cells respond poorly to organismal controls and their potentialities for development are severely restricted. The generality of neoplastic cells are not, however, completely anarchic and the growths that they form are not completely chaotic, indicating that such cells do respond, in part at least, to the influences that regulate normal cells within an organism. Even a rather elaborate organization of structure and function is quite consistent with the neoplastic state.

This, then, is briefly the bulk, if by no means the sum, of what has been learned over the past one and one-third centuries about the basic biological concepts that underlie our present knowledge of the tumor problem. However, a true understanding of that problem will require a precise experimental definition of the basic cellular mechanisms that are responsible for the continued abnormal and autonomous proliferation of tumor cells. The so-called oncogenic agents such as the carcinogenic chemicals as well as X rays and other forms of radiation can be dismissed from consideration in this regard for, while they are important in the initiation of tumors, they play no part in the continued abnormal growth of the tumor cells. A part or all of the genetic information present in certain of the oncogenic viruses, on the other hand, appears to be required continuously for the maintenance of the neoplastic state. Yet this knowledge in itself provides no clue whatsoever as to why such viral genomes urge the affected cells to grow in an essentially unregulated and autonomous manner. This is equally true of postulated genetic mechanisms such as, for example, somatic mutation at the nuclear gene level.

The tumor problem is, in its very essence, a dynamic problem of abnormal and autonomous cell growth and division. A rapidly growing fully autonomous tumor cell may, in fact, be described as a highly efficient proliferating system the energy of which is directed largely toward a synthesis of substances that are required specifically for continued cell growth and division. The transition from a normal resting cell to a tumor cell must, therefore, involve a radical reorientation in biosynthetic metabolism, going from the precisely regulated metabolism concerned with differentiated function to one involving an increased and continued synthesis of the nucleic acids, the mitotic and enzymatic proteins, as well as other substances required specifically for cell growth and division (501). It would appear, therefore, that an understanding of the tumor problem involves a characterization of the cellular mechanisms responsible for this major and persistent switch in biosynthetic metabolism. Statements found in the literature which question the validity of this concept will be commented on in Chapter VII.

It is the purpose of the present book to develop in detail and to document insofar as that is now possible the thesis that the tumor problem is fundamentally a problem of anomalous differentiation with the obvious implication that the heritable cellular change involved in tumorigenesis is similar in principle to that found in normal developmental processes. If that is true it would provide a unifying concept for the development of tumors generally.

CHAPTER II

The Regulation of Cell Division

The Normal Cell Cycle

Since the tumor problem is, in its very essence, a dynamic problem of abnormal and autonomous cell growth and division, it appears that any real understanding of the nature of neoplastic growth may have to await a genuine understanding of the nature of those mechanisms that regulate mitosis and division in normal cell types. The experimental oncologist is interested in persistently dividing cells and in discovering an explanation as to why neoplastic cells divide persistently. It would seem appropriate, therefore, to examine briefly what is known about regulatory mechanisms concerned in normal cell growth and division. The processes involved in cell division have now been studied in many different species of animals and plants. Although there are some differences in detail in the way cells of different organisms divide, it is striking to note how very similar the main features of cell division are from the unicellular algae and protozoa to flowering plants and vertebrates. For that reason, examples that have been used here to illustrate certain points have been taken from taxonomically very different types of organisms.

In any proliferating population of cells the individual members commonly go through a cell cycle that consists of the now familiar phases which are designated as G_1, S, G_2, M, and D. The G_1 phase denotes that portion of interphase prior to the onset of DNA synthesis. It is that period in the cell cycle in which there are a synthesis and mobilization of substrates and enzymes required for DNA synthesis. The G_1 phase is followed by a period of nuclear DNA replication which is known as the S phase. The G_2 phase, on the other hand, applies to the period between the end of nuclear DNA synthesis and just prior to the onset of mitosis. The mitotic process itself constitutes the M phase of the cell cycle. Typically, although by no means universally as evidenced by multinucleate cells, the end result of mitosis is the production of two daughter cells by a process known as cytokinesis. This represents the D phase of the cell cycle. The capacity of cells to regulate the sequence of events that culminate in cell division is apparent. It has, indeed, been suggested by Mazia (345) that a cell that does not divide is a cell that is blocked at some point in the cell cycle. What is known about the processes involved in cell division has been reviewed in detail (345, 500, 501, 39, 404, 479).

The process of cell division proceeds, then, through a continuously integrated series of closely related biochemical events beginning in early interphase and culminating in the division of one cell into two. Perhaps no event in the cell cycle is closer to being central to the initiation of mitosis and cell division than is the duplication of DNA. Once a cell starts to synthesize DNA it commonly, but not always, as evidenced by the G_2 phase block to be described later, proceeds through mitosis and cell division without interruption until the next G_1 phase is reached. This means, of course, that the decision as to whether a cell will divide is often made shortly before or during the transition from the G_1 to the S phase in the cell cycle. Since the regulation of mitosis and cell division in many instances is controlled by the initiation of DNA synthesis it would appear necessary, as a first step, to attempt to analyze events that lead to the synthesis of DNA.

G_1 and S Phases

It is during the G_1 phase of the cell cycle that a synthesis and mobilization of substrates and enzymes required for DNA synthesis take place. Ribonucleic acid and protein, but not nuclear DNA, are actively synthesized during that phase. Factors that may intervene in the regulation of DNA synthesis may be listed as (1) the presence of proper RNA and protein; (2) the availability of nucleotide pools; (3) the presence of DNA polymerase; (4) the ability to convert nonprimer DNA to the primer condition, i.e., to convert DNA into a form that permits its duplication; (5) the presence of a cytoplasmic initiator required for DNA synthesis.

The presence of proper RNA and protein, adequate nucleotide

pools, DNA polymerase, primer formation, and the presence of a cytoplasmic initiator are obviously essential if DNA synthesis is to occur. Questions of regulation, therefore, arise in this connection. Let us, then, consider briefly each of these essential components in order with the use of a few selected examples.

RNA and Protein. Hotta and Stern (244, 245, 246, 247), working with naturally synchronous cells of microsporogenous tissues of plants, used various inhibitors to study RNA and protein synthesis. These investigators found that *de novo* synthesis of protein takes place repeatedly during the mitotic and meiotic cycles and this is preceded by the production of RNA (presumably messenger RNA). Thus, these investigators suggested that the sequential activation of different genes responsible for the production of different RNA's and proteins takes place in different phases of the cell cycle and that this accounts for the direction and nature of the different macromolecular species that are synthesized. The differential activation of the genome with the resulting production of a new and specific macromolecular species is well illustrated with the use of thymidine kinase as a marker for new protein synthesis since that enzyme is easily measured quantitatively. Thymidine kinase is concerned with thymidine phosphorylation. The precise regulation of this enzyme during the cell cycle is shown in studies on sporogenous tissues of lily and trillium (244, 245). In the microspore of lily, interphase occupies a period of about 20 days. During this period thymidine kinase activity is found at significant levels for only about 12 to 16 hours or for approximately 5% of interphase time. This abrupt peak of enzyme activity is present about one day before DNA synthesis begins.

These studies illustrate very well, then, several aspects of the regulatory process. They show that enzyme activity appears very abruptly in the cell cycle and that enzyme synthesis arises *de novo*. The interval of enzyme synthesis is limited to 8 hours of a 20-day period of interphase after which time enzyme synthesis is stopped, and within a few hours thereafter enzyme activity within a cell reaches a very low level or disappears. Studies that bear on the question of the differential activation of the genome with the resulting production of new species of RNA and protein during the cell cycle are considered in greater detail in the last chapter of this book.

Precursor Pools. Adequate nucleotide pools are obviously essential for DNA synthesis. One may reasonably ask, therefore, how the precursor pool is regulated and whether pool size has any effect on the initiation of DNA synthesis. Available evidence suggests that precursor pools are regulated with respect to formation and utilization. Deoxyribonucleotides required for nuclear DNA synthesis do not appear to be produced in significant amounts during all periods of the cell cycle. It is clear, moreover, that deoxyribonucleotides are not accumulated in nonproliferating cells in the absence of DNA synthesis. There is, in fact, evidence for the periodic accumulation and removal of precursors in naturally occurring synchronous cells such as those found in microsporogenous tissues of plants (478). Thus, in certain kinds of cells at least, the evidence is clear that the initiation of DNA synthesis is correlated with the synthesis of enzyme-mediated precursor formation.

Other types of evidence bear on this question. Embryos of germinating wheat seeds synthesize large amounts of the enzyme thymidine kinase. If, however, the endosperm is removed from the embryo, enzyme synthesis stops abruptly. Synthesis of the enzyme is again resumed if a solution containing thymidine is added to the embryos. The rate of resumption of enzyme synthesis is dependent upon the level of exogenous thymidine added to the system, as is the rate of DNA synthesis (248). Here, then, we have a simple example of thymidine level controlling the periodicity of DNA synthesis by limiting the over-all reaction rate. Thus a mechanism for controlling the net rate of deoxyribonucleotide production appears to exist. This does not, of course, mean that such control necessarily encompasses the essence of reproductive regulation.

In the ciliated protozoon *Tetrahymena* there is evidence that the precursor pool is replenished only during the S phase of the cell cycle. If cells of this protozoon are deprived of an essential amino acid, which stops all protein synthesis within a few minutes, at any time between cell division and the beginning of DNA synthesis, the next cell division will not occur. If, on the other hand, the essential amino acid is withheld at any time after the beginning of DNA synthesis, the next cell division will invariably take place. It is clear from those experiments that some amino acid-dependent event essential for the completion of the cell cycle occurs at the transition between the G_1 and S phases. It has been found, moreover, that deprivation of the essential amino acid between cell division and DNA synthesis does not prevent the initiation of DNA synthesis. DNA increases about 20% but no more under those conditions. The cells are unable to utilize an exogenous source of tritiated thymidine for the synthesis of this 20% increase in DNA although thymidine is normally readily taken up and incorporated by those cells.

To attempt to explain the results of those experiments the synthesis and destruction of the enzyme thymidine kinase were studied. It was found that without the essential amino acid the cell was unable to synthesize the enzyme at the transition between the G_1 and S phases and the labeled thymidine in the medium was not utilized. However, the pre-existing nucleotide pools are utilized for DNA synthesis and such synthesis stops when those pools are exhausted, at a time when about 20% increase in DNA is achieved. If the cells of *Tetrahymena* are allowed to make the G_1-to-S transition before they are deprived of the essential amino acid, DNA synthesis goes to completion and labeled thymidine in the medium is taken up by the cells and incorporated into their DNA. The implication of these experiments is, therefore, that thymidine kinase is synthesized at the beginning of S phase and is destroyed when S phase is completed. This interpretation of the observed results is supported by the fact that *Tetrahymena* cells do not take up labeled thymidine into the precursor pool during the non-S phases of the cell cycle although such a pool apparently exists during the entire cycle. The pool appears, then, to be replenished only during the S phase. The results of these experiments clearly indicate that protein synthesis is not necessary for the initiation of DNA synthesis although newly synthesized protein is required for the maintenance of DNA synthesis in *Tetrahymena*.

Baserga et al. (40), working with Ehrlich ascites tumor cells, have reported the presence of an actinomycin D-sensitive step in the G_1 phase of the cell cycle which precedes DNA synthesis. This block prevents the cells from entering S phase. Small amounts of actinomycin D do not, on the other hand, inhibit DNA synthesis, the G_2 phase, or mitosis if the cells are in a stage of the cell cycle beyond the antibiotic-sensitive step when that material is applied. Since small concentrations of actinomycin D are considered to be specific inhibitors of DNA-dependent RNA synthesis, the results would suggest that the actinomycin D-sensitive step in the G_1 phase is concerned with the synthesis of one or more kinds of ribonucleic acid. The studies showed, in fact, that it was the synthesis of ribosomal RNA that was largely inhibited by actinomycin D in this system. The activities of thymidine kinase and DNA polymerase were not affected. The important conclusions that arise from these and many other similar studies are that there are a number of critical points in the cell cycle which are characterized by an increased sensitivity to various agents. The establishment of these critical points in the cell cycle by virtue of their increased sensitivity to specific inhibitors led to Mazia's (345) concept of "points of no return" in which a metabolic block, once overcome, leads to insensitivity of subsequent phases to inhibitors that had disrupted some prior event in the cell cycle.

DNA Polymerase. The polymerization of deoxyriboside triphosphates into DNA raises some interesting questions. In certain organisms such as *Euplotes,* DNA polymerase is apparently present throughout the cell cycle including non-DNA-synthesizing periods (285). In contrast, in rabbit kidney cortex cells Lieberman et al. (306) found that DNA polymerase and thymidine kinase increase only at the time that DNA synthesis begins. However, in synchronized cultures of L cells DNA polymerase activity increases when DNA synthesis is inhibited and decreases when DNA synthesis is allowed to continue (204). Yet, according to Stern (479) these issues should not be treated naively by simply asking whether the polymerase is always present or whether it is induced at the appropriate time in the cell cycle. He points out that the intimate juxtaposition of the enzyme and the DNA filament at once involves the problem of structural features of what have been called "starting points." Unequivocal evidence obtained through autoradiographic studies has led to the conclusion that highly localized control of the initiation of DNA replication exists. Each chromosome has several starting regions of DNA replication and these regions are fixed characteristics of the species (309). This matter has been discussed in detail by Taylor (505). Thus, even if it is assumed that each chromosome contains a single DNA filament, that filament must be interrupted in some distinctive way by a number of starting regions.

In addition to the problem of "starting points," Mueller and his associates (366) have found that within the same nucleus DNA may exist in two physiological states. Using synchronized cultures of HeLa cells together with appropriate antibiotics, these workers found that in one of these states DNA is competent and capable of rapid replication while in the other an additional stimulus in the form of a protein is needed in order for the DNA to acquire competence for replication. The synthesis of this protein, in turn, is triggered by the action of so-called synchronizers (366, 498). Mueller (365) has shown, then, that cells which begin DNA synthesis require additional *de novo* synthesis of RNA and protein without which they cannot achieve the subsequent stages of DNA synthesis in the chromosomes.

Cytoplasmic Initiator of DNA Synthesis. Recent studies have indicated that intrachromosomal regulation of DNA synthesis takes place against a background of a more general type of intracellular regulation. If that is true, then one would expect that nuclei sharing the same cytoplasm would divide at the same time. Koller (293) has indicated that synchrony is, in fact, the rule in the case of multinucleate tumor cells, megakaryocytes of human bone, cells of growing root tips, and spermatocytes of insects and of mammals.

Further studies designed to elucidate at a biological level the cellular mechanisms that regulate DNA synthesis during the cell cycle have strongly implicated cytoplasmic factors as initiators of that process. de Terra (149), using the large ciliate *Stentor coeruleus* as the test object, transplanted nuclei of G_1 and D phase cells into the cytoplasm of S phase cells and found that such nuclei began to synthesize DNA. Conversely, when nuclei of S phase cells were transplanted into cytoplasm of G_1 and D phase cells, DNA synthesis was inhibited. The results of these studies, together with those reported by Prescott and Goldstein (405) using *Amoeba proteus* cells, may be interpreted either in terms of cytoplasmic inhibitors of DNA synthesis which are present in non-S phase cells but absent in S cells or in terms of cytoplasmic initiators which are found in S phase cells but are absent in non-S cells. The initiator concept, which was initially put forward by Jacob et al. (260) in the *Escherichia coli* system, appears to apply because when S and G_1 *Stentor* cells of equal size are grafted together DNA synthesis is initiated in the G_1 cell, not inhibited in the S cell. de Terra (148) believes, moreover, that all of the major nuclear events in the cell cycle of *Stentor* studied thus far are under cytoplasmic control.

Nucleocytoplasmic interactions of the type described above are not restricted to protozoa. It was found that nuclei from gastrula endoderm cells of the frog as well as from adult liver, brain, and blood cells synthesized DNA following their injection into normal frog egg cytoplasm. In the case of liver, brain, and blood cell nuclei this constitutes a significant change in function because not more than 1% of the nuclei in those cells normally incorporate tritiated thymidine in periods of time used in those studies. It was found, moreover, that the method used to prepare such nuclei did not in itself induce DNA synthesis. The change in nuclear function, in this instance, was induced by exposing the mature nuclei to normal unfertilized egg cytoplasm. The cytoplasmic influence was not class-specific since over 90% of mouse liver nuclei were also induced to synthesize DNA when injected into frog eggs.

In a continuation of those studies Gurdon et al. (219, 210) implanted nuclei from adult frog brain cells into unfertilized frog eggs. Although these nuclei do not support normal development, they respond to egg cytoplasm by DNA synthesis as do transplanted embryonic nuclei which do support normal development. These experiments demonstrated further that the state of egg cytoplasm which induces DNA synthesis is completely absent from oocytes, the cells which mature into eggs. It has been found, moreover, that this cytoplasmic state arises as an effect of pituitary hormone on mature oocytes. The induction of DNA synthesis cannot, however, be explained solely as a direct effect of the hormone on the injected nuclei because DNA synthesis is not induced during incubation of isolated nuclei to which the hormone has been added.

Cytoplasmic control over nucleic acid biosynthesis has also been demonstrated in heterokaryons resulting from cell fusion (228) as well as in embryos of *Rana pipiens* (87).

In all of the cases cited above it appears that an appropriate cytoplasm can exert a positive inducing effect on inactive nuclei. The same positive control was recently observed by Thompson and McCarthy (513) with the use of isolated nuclei *in vitro*. In this instance resting nuclei from mouse liver cells or hen erythrocytes were used. The addition of mouse liver cytoplasm had little effect while cytoplasm from rapidly growing ascites or L cells caused an immediate increase in the rate of synthesis of the nucleic acids. The activity of the stimulatory factors found in the cytoplasm appeared to be correlated with the rate of nucleic acid biosynthesis in the cells from which the cytoplasm was derived. The stimulatory factor(s) is neither species- nor order-specific. A partial purification of the cytoplasmic factor that stimulates DNA synthesis has shown it to be a heat-stable molecule which can be distinguished from cytoplasmic DNA polymerase. This factor withstands repeated freezing and thawing, while an RNA stimulating cytoplasmic factor is also thermostable but is inactivated by repeated freezing and thawing.

Before passing to the G_2 phase it should be noted that not all cellular DNA synthesis occurs during the S phase. The studies of Parsons (389) and of Evans (173) indicate that mitochondrial DNA is not synthesized during the S phase of the cell cycle.

It may be concluded, therefore, as a generalization, that DNA synthesis, viewed as a marker for the doubling of the chromosome substance, is a normal feature of the pathway to cell division. Cells which will not divide do not usually increase their DNA content while, on the other hand, cells that have doubled their DNA need not necessarily divide.

It is clear, moreover, from this brief review of selected examples presented above that the regulation of DNA synthesis is a complex process that may be controlled at many points in the cell cycle by many different factors. It would, nevertheless, appear that under the usual circumstances the prime factor that determines whether or not DNA synthesis proceeds is the presence or absence of a cytoplasmic initiator of that process. The regulation of a cytoplasmic initiator of the type described above could very well represent a fundamental point of departure between a normal cell and a tumor cell. Although one would expect that cytoplasmic factor to be found in any dividing cell population whether normal or tumor, it may well be that fundamental regulatory differences exist when the cells are growing *in situ*.

G_2 Phase

The G_2 phase, like the G_1 phase of the cell cycle, is a period of protein and RNA synthesis. Since these two phases occupy different positions in the cell cycle with respect to DNA synthesis and mitosis, it is clear that protein and RNA synthesis must be basically different in certain specific and essential respects in the two phases.

Although as indicated earlier, most cells are arrested in the G_1 phase, Gelfant (196) has shown that certain mouse ear epidermal cells may, in fact, be blocked in the G_2 phase from which they enter nuclear division directly after suitable stimulation. It was found that a single layer of mouse ear epidermal cells can be subdivided into distinct and separate cell types which differ in their patterns of behavior during the cell division cycle or in their physiological requirements for mitosis. Gelfant found that two major cell types exist within the basal layer of epidermis. These were named the G_1 and G_2 epidermal cell populations. The G_1 cell populations moved through the cell cycle in the usual manner. Mitosis is first initiated in these cells from the G_1 period as evidenced by the fact that the stimulated cells of this population enter the S phase, incorporate thymidine H^3, move through G_2, and appear as labeled mitoses in autoradiographs. The G_2 cell populations, on the other hand, have an extraordinarily long G_2 period and mitosis is initiated from that period of the cycle. When cells of this population are stimulated experimentally they do not incorporate thymidine H^3 because they are in a post-DNA synthesis period. Among the major G_2 category of cells Gelfant (197) presented evidence for the existence of separate sugar-responding, sodium ion-responding, and potassium ion-responding epidermal cells. These physiological subpopulations display their specific physiological requirements for mitosis during the G_2 period of the cell cycle. It has been indicated (198) that discrete G_1 and G_2 cell populations exist in a wide variety of both plant and animal tissues.

That a block to DNA synthesis occurs in the G_2 phase as well as the G_1 phase of amoeba was conclusively demonstrated by the studies of Prescott and Goldstein referred to above. These investigators transplanted S phase nuclei into G_2 phase cytoplasm and found that DNA synthesis in the nuclei was arrested. The reciprocal transplantation resulted in an active DNA synthesis by G_2 nuclei placed in S phase cytoplasm. They favored the view that an initiator of DNA synthesis was present in S phase cytoplasm but absent in G_2 cytoplasm of the amoeba.

It is interesting to note that under the influence of chemical carcinogens such as 4-dimethylaminoazobenzene (DAB) hepatic cells of rats cease to respond to the mitotic stimulus of partial hepatectomy. Banerjee (28) found that while there was very little increase in the mitotic index of liver tissue after partial hepatectomy during azo-dye hepatocarcinogenesis, there was a significant increase in the frequency of the labeled cells as compared with those in the nonhepatectomized controls. These results were interpreted to mean that the hepatocytes stimulated by partial hepatectomy did synthesize DNA but did not proceed further in the mitotic cycle where they were arrested at the G_2 phase.

Simard, Cousineau, and Daoust (453a) studied azo-dye hepatocarcinogenesis in the rat and found that the neoplastic transformation was associated with an elimination or inhibition of both G_1 and G_2 blocks in the cell cycle. These changes contributed to the acceleration of cell proliferation at the sites of tumor formation.

M Phase

When the nucleus of a cell enters mitotic division it commits itself to complete structural reorganization. The chromosomes condense into compact structures and a faithful replication and precise distribution of the genetic material occur. The nuclear membrane disappears or is profoundly changed. The nucleolus is commonly broken down while other nonchromosomal contents of the nucleus including the RNA's are lost to the cytoplasm. Thus, following mitosis, the chromosomes appear to begin again with a clean slate. It has, in fact, been suggested that mitosis may be a mechanism whereby a cell destroys its nuclear history so that in order for a cell to reprogram its information, it must pass through a mitotic cycle. According to this idea, the processes of normal differentiation and neoplastic transformation would be impossible without mitotic division. That there may, in fact, be some validity to that notion is suggested by results of recent studies on normal differentiation of plant (186) and animal (see Chapter V) cells as well as in neoplastic transformations in the plant and animal fields. All three of the non-self-limiting neoplastic diseases of plants described here require irritation accompanying a wound with resulting cell division in order to fix the tumorous state in a cell. Similarly, tumor cell transformations resulting from X-irradiation (64), carcinogenic chemicals (51), and viruses (517) have been found to require cell replication to fix the transformed state in the animal cell.

Not only do profound changes in the nucleus occur during the M phase of the cell cycle but the mitochondria may also undergo a number of changes and some may disappear, while the endoplasmic reticulum may lose its characteristic structure. There is a loss of polysomes with a resulting decrease in protein synthesis. The ribosomes that are present are largely inactive but amino acid incorporating activity may be restored *in vitro* by exposing such ribosomes to low concentrations of trypsin (440). Even the surface structure changes in certain types of cells such as in amoebae or in fibroblasts, which normally are irregular in shape but become spherical when they enter division. The most conspicuous feature of an M phase cell is the mitotic spindle which is sometimes huge and may occupy much of the interior of a cell.

Methods for isolating the mitotic apparatus from cells have made possible a chemical characterization of the spindle fiber material (346). In the initial studies Mazia and Dan showed that the spindle in dividing sea urchin eggs is formed from distinct protein, whose amino acid composition was determined. Electrophoretic studies showed two fast-moving components, one of which was present in large and the other in much smaller amounts. Ultracentrifugation studies indicated a molecular weight of about 45,000 for the most abundant component. Further studies by Mazia and Roslansky (347) showed that an isolated mitotic figure contained about 11% of the total protein of dividing sea urchin egg cells. Swann (501) suggests that the mitotic apparatus may constitute between one-fourth and one-half of the dry weight of certain somatic cells. It is clear, therefore, that a cell entering division must either synthesize a large amount of new protein or must assemble the mitotic apparatus from protein already present before division occurs. It is important to recognize that in either case new synthesis amounting to a doubling of the mitotic apparatus proteins must occur in each cell cycle. The spindle fiber protein is, moreover, a specialized protein which has a highly special-ized function to perform. A second major property of the spindle mechanism is polarity. The spindle apparatus has poles and chromo-some movements are polar.

At and before the turn of the present century cytologists Boveri (69) and Strasburger (496) postulated that cells contained a distinct fibrous component which was randomly distributed before division but which was assembled and became oriented into the mitotic apparatus at the time of division. That spindle fiber protein was present in a cell prior to division was first clearly demonstrated by immunochemical methods (549, 550, 551). It was found in those studies that an extract of unfertilized sea urchin eggs contained at least one antigen that matched that of the dissolved isolated mitotic apparatus, while the dissolved apparatus yielded no antigens that were not present in the unfertilized egg. This led to the conclusion that the protein of the mitotic apparatus is synthesized before nuclear division and is merely assembled at the time of division. Shortly thereafter, Ledbetter and Porter (301) found, with the use of the electron microscope, a microtubular system in both plant and animal cells which is now believed to represent the building blocks from which the spindle fibers and centrioles develop.

Spindle fibers, then, appear to be composed of parallel arrays of microtubules or thin filaments which are formed by a reversible association of globular protein molecules. The spindle fibers are labile structures and are not stably aligned and cross-linked. These structures exist, moreover, in a dynamic equilibrium together with a large pool of unassociated molecules. The assembly of molecules with the resulting formation of filaments is believed to be controlled by the activities of orienting centers and concentrations of active pool material. Inoué and Sato (256) have recently hypothesized that spindle fibers do not elongate and contract by folding and unfolding of polypeptide chains in the protein molecule but rather that they elongate by the addition and alignment of molecules which contribute to a pushing action, while the fibers shorten and pull the chromosomes to the poles as protein molecules are removed from the filaments.

Recent studies on the chemistry of the microtubules are not in complete agreement as to the size of the basic unit. Sakai (439) and Kiefer et al. (284) have isolated a 2.5S protein from the mitotic apparatus of sea urchin eggs with a particle weight of about 34,000. Kane (271), on the other hand, has obtained a 22S protein from isolated mitotic apparatuses as well as from whole sea urchin eggs. The protein is monodispersed and has a particle weight of 880,000. It can be dissociated into subunits of 110,000 particle weight. Stephens (477) has studied some physical and chemical properties of this protein. He has found that the 22S protein obtained either from unfertilized eggs or from the isolated mitotic apparatus shows identical amino acid compositions. The 22S material makes up more than 90% of the KCl soluble proteins of the spindle. Its concentration in the spindle parallels spindle birefringence and correlates with the number of microtubules during D_2O treatment. It appears, therefore, to be a likely candidate for the spindle fiber protein. Nevertheless, the 2.5S protein described by Kiefer et al. (284) would appear to have a dimension better fitting the electron microscope periodicity seen in the microtubules of the spindle. It is not yet clear whether these are two different and distinct proteins or whether they are the same protein polymerized to different degrees. The important point for the discussion which follows is that a new and highly specialized protein is synthesized in very significant amounts during each cell cycle.

D Phase

Cytokinesis is clearly a facultative end point of mitosis, as evidenced by the rather common occurrence in both the animal and plant kingdoms of multinucleate cells in which mitosis has occurred without corresponding cell division. Typically, however, cytokinesis follows mitosis. It is, nevertheless, possible to dissociate the processes of mitosis and cell division experimentally in a number of ways. X-ray-induced cellular giantism with the resulting production of polyploid cells containing one or more nuclei has been reported in egg cells, spermatocytes, corneal cells, grasshopper neuroblasts, plant cells, and mammalian cells. The production of such multinucleate giant cells is commonly associated with a failure of the cell division mechanism although it may also result from cell fusion. That such a mechanism may be based in the cytoplasm is suggested by the studies of Daniels (139) who grafted unirradiated cytoplasm of the giant amoeba *Pelomyxa carolinensis* to cells in which division had been blocked by ultraviolet or X-irradiation. It was found in those studies that the presence of a bit of grafted unirradiated cytoplasm reversed the inhibition and completely repaired the radiation-induced damage.

Adler et al. (5) studied a mutant of *Escherichia coli* that was characterized by a failure to complete cytokinesis. Cell growth and nuclear division were unimpaired and long nonseptate multinuclear filaments were formed. These filaments did not divide unless they were treated with a cytokinesis-stimulating substance. Such a substance was isolated from an extract of normal *E. coli* cells. That substance is apparently a polypeptide. In addition, two other factors were found in the extract. One of these, a low molecular weight compound, inhibits cytokinesis while the other, associated with 100S ribosome fraction, balances the activity of the stimulator and inhibitor.

In higher plant species the processes of cell enlargement and cell division are controlled by the quantitative interaction of two growth-regulating hormones, the auxins and the cytokinins. The auxins are concerned with cell enlargement while the cytokinins act synergistically with the auxins to promote cell division. If, for example, a fragment of tobacco pith parenchyma tissue is isolated and planted on a simple chemically defined culture medium containing mineral salts, sucrose, and three vitamins, the pith cells neither enlarge nor divide but remain quiescent indefinitely. If, now, that medium is supplemented with an auxin (indoleacetic acid) at a concentration of 1 ppm, the pith cells enlarge greatly in size but they do not divide. DNA synthesis proceeds so that such cells become polyploid and may contain one to many nuclei. If, in addition to an auxin, a cytokinin such as kinetin (6-furfurylaminopurine) or a naturally occurring cell division factor (572) is added to the medium at a concentration of 0.5 ppm, a profuse growth accompanied by cell division results. It is thus possible in this system to delimit under precisely defined experimental conditions cell enlargement accompanied by DNA synthesis and mitosis, on the one hand, and mitosis accompanied by cytokinesis, on the other (259) (see Fig. 3).

Stevens and associates have described an interesting case in which the incidence of multinucleate cells reaches 25% in a hamster ascites tumor (482). It was found that the level of multinucleation could be significantly decreased *in vivo* and *in vitro* by estrogens. However, when the tumor cells were washed and cultured in a defined medium, estrogens were ineffective (480). It was subsequently found that when small amounts of ascites fluid or serum from cancer-bearing hamsters but not normal serum was added to the culture medium, the corrective effect of estrogens on multinucleation was reinstated. Janus green B and 2,4-dinitrophenol abolish that effect. Recent studies (481) have shown that thymidine 5'triphosphate or thymidine 5'monophosphate induces cytokinesis, while other nucleotides are ineffective in

A   B

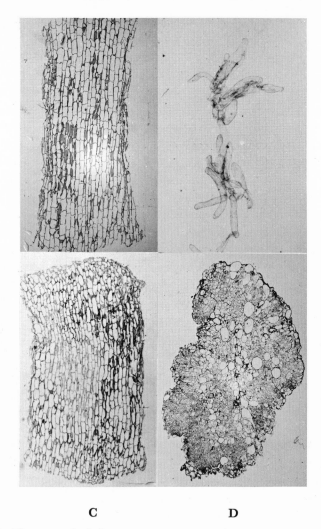

C   D

Fig. 3. The control of the processes of cell enlargement and cell division in tobacco pith parenchyma cells with the use of an auxin (naphthalene-acetic acid) and a cytokinin (6-furfurylaminopurine). Histological sections of: **A.** Untreated control. **B.** Treated with auxin at a concentration of 1 mg/l; note cells have enlarged greatly in size without dividing. **C.** Treated with a cytokinin at a concentration of 0.5 mg/l; this compound does not promote either cell enlargement or cell division. **D.** Treated with both an auxin (1 mg/l) and a cytokinin (0.5 mg/l). A rapid growth accompanied by cell division results from the synergistic effect of the two growth-regulating substances.

that respect. The administration of malonate or of oxalacetate, on the other hand, causes an increased number of multinucleate cells. Of interest here is the finding that thymidine 5′triphosphate or thymidine 5′monophosphate causes cytokinesis to occur in multinucleate cells without estrogen, while serum from cancer-bearing hamsters or bradykinin has the same effect only in the presence of estrogens. Stevens has suggested that cytokinesis in this system may be controlled through the usual oxidative phosphorylating mechanisms in a cell. Bradykinin or cancer serum and estrogen overcome this defect probably by an alternative route leading to the synthesis of a substance(s) necessary for cytokinesis.

The attempt that has been made above to sketch out a number of events in the cell cycle which appear to be concerned with the total process of new cell reproduction has clearly indicated that there are many potential and several major points at which the cycle may be interrupted. It has, in fact, been suggested (345) that it might be constructive to look upon every cell that does not divide as a cell that is blocked at some point on the pathway to division. The implication of that statement is, of course, that most cells, even highly differentiated ones, with few notable exceptions, are capable of dividing under the proper conditions. A further and, as far as the present discussion is concerned, a most important implication of that statement is that in persistently dividing cells, such as those found in true tumors as well as in normal cell culture, and in most unicellular organisms, all of the naturally occurring blocks in the cell cycle have been removed, thus enabling such cells to divide continuously in an otherwise suitable environment.

Other Regulatory Mechanisms

In the examples presented above all of the major blocks in the cell cycle appear to depend on the absence of some essential factor rather than on the presence of an inhibitory substance. Yet, naturally occurring organ-specific substances inhibitory to cell division have been extracted by Saetren (436, 437) from liver and kidney. Similar substances have been isolated by Rytömaa and Kiviniemi (434) from granulocytes and by Bullough and Laurence (100) from mouse ear epidermal cells. The last-mentioned investigators have demonstrated that cell division in mouse ear epidermal cells is regulated by an unstable complex of an epidermal chalone and adrenalin. This conclusion was based on finding that epidermal cell division is strongly inhibited by adrenalin and this fact, according to Bullough (98), forms the basis of the well-known diurnal mitotic rhythm found in epidermal cells.

It was also observed that the antimitotic activity of adrenalin is tissue-specific and not mitotic-specific since active hair bulbs and rectal mucosa as well as many other cell types are not affected by it. This finding suggested to Bullough that epidermal cells contain a specific factor with which adrenalin reacts and thus exerts its antimitotic activity. Such a factor, which is synthesized by epidermal cells and which diffuses slowly from such cells especially in the region of a wound, was isolated. Water extracts of macerated epidermal cells of mice were effective in suppressing mitosis both *in vitro* and *in vivo* when epidermal cells of mice were used as the experimental test object. Extracts similarly made from a wide variety of other tissues had no effect when tested on mouse ear epidermal cells. Thus, the chalone appears to be tissue-specific but not a species-specific substance.

The epidermal chalone has now been isolated and partially characterized chemically. It has been found to be a basic glycoprotein having a molecular weight of about 35,000 (243a).

The evidence indicates that neither the chalone nor the adrenalin is able to function effectively alone and that in the normal epidermis they act together to regulate cell division. Bullough (99) has suggested that this complex acts somehow to control gene expression. Here, then, is a homeostatic mechanism that is based on inhibition rather than on specific stimulation. Yet it is well known that a number of hormones and, more particularly, the estrogens exert a profound stimulatory effect on mitotic activity in target tissues of mammals. Bullough has interpreted such findings as involving a neutralization of the inhibitory effects of the chalone by the mitogenic hormones. The results reported thus far do not, moreover, preclude the possibility that specific stimulators of mitosis and division are synthesized by the cell following removal of the chalone. An antichalone has, in fact, been isolated from serum and has been shown to stimulate division of granulocytes and to play an important role in the control of granulocyte production (435). This substance acts in the cell cycle prior to nuclear DNA synthesis. It would thus appear that concepts of specific stimuli versus specific inhibitors as regulators of cell division need not necessarily be mutually exclusive. Aside from the so-called mitogenic hormones there are, of course, many different naturally occurring substances that directly affect the regulation of growth in mammals. Among these might be mentioned promine and retine (503), the nerve growth factor (305) and the skin factor (123), the mammalian cell growth protein, fetuin (409), and many others.

Of particular interest in this regard are results that have recently been reported with the use of the 3T3 line of mouse fibroblast cells. Todaro, Lazar, and Green (519) have studied the effect of serum on cell division in this system and have indicated that a factor(s) present in serum is required for cell division. Viral transformed 3T3 cells have, interestingly enough, a greatly reduced requirement for that factor(s). Attempts to isolate and characterize the serum factor(s) have recently been carried out by Holley and Kiernan (241). Biologically very active compounds were isolated not only from serum but from urine as well. The serum factor appears to be a protein having a molecular weight of about 100,000. The material from urine, on the other hand, has a significantly lower molecular weight, is inactivated by pronase, but is relatively stable to heat at 100°C. It is biologically active at microgram levels. A number of commercial preparations of hormones including ACTH, follicle-stimulating hormone, insulin, luteinizing hormone, gonadotropin, growth hormone, oxytocin, and prolactin were assayed and found to be biologically inactive in this system.

Temin (510, 511) has found that an insulin-like factor in serum is required for cell division by cultured chick cells. Transformation of cultured chick cells by Rous sarcoma virus lowers the requirement for this serum factor.

It may be more profitable for the purposes of this discussion to examine the broader question of how such inhibitors or stimulators of cell division exert their effects in cells at a biological level. Swann (501) has argued most persuasively that what is commonly called a mitogenic stimulus, involving either removal of inhibitors or addition of stimulators, marks the beginning of an entirely new pattern of synthesis in a cell and very probably the temporary cessation of the previous pattern of synthesis concerned with differentiated function.

When the effects of the mitogenic stimulus are terminated there is normally a reversal of those effects. The new pattern of synthesis that is characteristic of a dividing cell must involve a major switch in biosynthetic metabolism. The most obvious product synthesized by a cell preparing to divide is the new protein that is found in the mitotic apparatus. This, as indicated above, is a highly specialized protein that has a highly specialized function to perform. It constitutes 11% of the total protein in sea urchin eggs and perhaps as much as 30% or more of the protein present in certain tumor cells.

It thus becomes clear that proteins concerned with the division process account for a significant part of the total components of a dividing cell. Synthesis of such protein is carried out largely in lieu of synthesis of the specialized proteins that are concerned with differentiated function and are found in normal resting cells. Thus, an entirely new pattern of synthesis is initiated in a dividing cell. Swann has argued that a switch of biosynthetic pattern of this type is in every way comparable to the switches involved in the process of induction by which cellular differentiation is brought about in the course of development. If, as appears likely, that is true, then the commonly recognized antagonism between cell differentiation and cell division is understandable. Nevertheless, there appears at first sight to be a significant difference between "induction" of division in a normal cell, which is readily reversible (although this does not apply to the tumor cell), and the usual types of embryonic induction in which an inducer operates for a short time and initiates a new pattern of synthesis which is then more or less permanent.

Experiments such as those described by Jacoby, Trowell, and Willmer (263) suggest that the cell division stimulus present in embryo extract is effective only for a single cell generation. Using chick heart fibroblasts as the test object, these workers showed that embryo extract had to be added for less than one hour to produce a crop of mitoses some 10 to 20 hours later. The addition of embryo extract following the first burst of mitoses had no effect until some 16 hours later when a second crop of cell divisions occurred in those cells that had completed division earlier. It thus appears that the essential factor(s) in the embryo extract is required to be taken up for only a short period of time, many hours before cell division itself occurs. The cells then complete one division, after which time they become quiescent again unless they are stimulated with embryo extract to divide a second time. This, according to Swann, is exactly what one would expect of an inductive mechanism. The inducer should act for a short period of time, initiate a new pattern of synthesis, and thereafter have no effect. Indeed, if such an effect lasted for more than a few generations it would result in hyperplasia and, if long lasting, in neoplasia.

The essence of Swann's argument is, then, (1) that cell division is an inductive process similar to that involved in cell differentiation, and (2) that it is an expensive one as far as the economy of the cell is concerned, with the synthesis of new protein required for the mitotic apparatus accounting for much of the budget.

If it is accepted that the process of cell proliferation requires a radical reorientation of biosynthetic metabolism involving the very extensive synthesis of new and specialized protein which makes up a significant bulk of the cell mass, then it may be instructive to examine the problem of tumor growth from that point of view.

CHAPTER III

The Development of a
Capacity for Autonomous Growth

The Establishment of a New Pattern of Synthesis

The transformation of a normal cell into a tumor cell in both the animal and the plant fields clearly involves a profound switch in biosynthetic metabolism going from the precisely regulated metabolism concerned with differentiated function, which is characteristic of a normal resting cell, to one involving the persistently increased synthesis of the nucleic acids and the mitotic and enzymatic proteins as well as other substances that are specifically concerned with continued cell growth and division. A rapidly growing fully autonomous tumor cell may, in fact, be described as a highly efficient proliferating system the energy of which is directed largely toward a synthesis of substances required specifically for cell growth and division. This pattern of synthesis results in the complete or partial exclusion of proteins normally synthesized for purposes of differentiated function. It is not surprising to find, therefore, that rapidly growing fully autonomous tumor cells may show such a pronounced deterioration of form and function that it is often difficult for a pathologist to determine the precise cell type from which the tumor originated. This does not, of course, necessarily mean that the factors determining the pattern of synthesis concerned with differentiated function are lost in such cell types; they may simply be overwhelmed and, hence, not be expressed.

Such extreme dedifferentiation is not the general rule, however. Most tumors retain a sufficient capacity for differentiation and function so that they are readily identifiable as to the cell type of their origin and yet possess a capacity for autonomous growth. At the other extreme in this spectrum is found the fastidious metabolism associated with the normal resting cell. It thus appears that two areas of metabolism, the primitive of the tumor which is concerned with persistent cell division and the fastidious of the normal which is involved in differentiated function, compete with one another for ascendancy in a cell, and the degree to which a cell is transformed would appear to determine the extent to which either pattern is expressed. This, then, leads to the very fundamental question as to how these metabolic patterns are established and how a cell acquires a capacity for autonomous growth. In order to attempt to answer those questions attention must again be directed toward the factors that normally regulate cell growth and division. Despite much speculation, very little definitive information concerning these matters, particularly as they relate to the basic mechanisms underlying autonomous growth, is as yet available in the animal tumor field.

Autonomy in Animal Tumors

In attempting to account for the autonomous growth of animal tumor cells, Leo Loeb (318, 319) stated on the basis of his long experience in experimental cancer research:

Tentatively it may be assumed that . . . a growth substance is produced or increased in quantity in the cells and that the production of this substance is renewed autokatalytically. Thus growth processes of certain cells are intensified irreversibly and certain cellular, metabolic and functional processes are altered.

Similarly, Rous (425) has written:

Are there simple chemical agents which could be responsible for all these phenomena? The answer has long been available. In 1906 Bernard Fischer . . . injected substances of many sorts directly beneath the epidermis of rabbits in a search for one that might be responsible for cancers; and he hit upon a fat-soluble dye, Scharlach R, which caused the epithelial cells directly exposed to it to look and behave for the time being precisely as if they were carcinomatous. They multiplied actively, invaded the underlying tissue deeply, and even entered blood and lymph vessels. . . .

Fischer's failure to cause real cancers is our gain in the present connection, since he found that the cells which mimicked malignancy reverted completely to the normal as the Scharlach R disappeared from the site of injection. . . .

Rous continued:

Were substances with effects generally resembling those of Scharlach R, but differing in particulars, formed continually by some of the viruses accompanying animal cells [present author's insert: or by the cells under the influence of a virus], this would account for the entire gamut of the tumors.

The experiments of George and Eva Klein (289) dealing with the evolution of independence from stimulatory and inhibitory effects in tumors also appear to bear on this question. It was found that a number of ascites tumors which were originally hormone-dependent but transplanted often enough to have achieved apparently complete autonomy, do nevertheless show signs of hormone-dependence if administered in small inocula. These workers suggest that the cells "gradually acquire the ability . . . to produce and utilize endogenous substances capable of acting as substitutes for the exogenous stimuli previously needed. With a small cell number, such cell products may become too diluted and fall below an effective level, thereby making the cells once more dependent on the previously needed exogenous stimulus."

Bullough (99), on the other hand, has recently considered the effects of a permanent breakdown of the homeostatic mechanism based on the chalone-adrenalin complex in epidermal cells in relation to the cancer problem. Such a mechanism should, theoretically at least, offer a very simple and direct explanation for the development of a capacity for autonomous growth of epidermal cell types. In such a system one would need only to postulate the inability of a cell or cells to synthesize the epidermal chalone in order to account for the continued unregulated and autonomous proliferation of those cells. Conversely, the loss of the ability to regulate the processes of division in cells that do not synthesize chalone should again be repaired and the division process brought under control by supplying such cells continually with an exogenous source of the chalone in the presence of adrenalin.

Since the epidermal chalone is a tissue-specific substance, it would appear that such an approach would offer an almost ideal method for the suppression of tumors of epidermal origin. Bullough and Laurence (101) have, in fact, claimed some degree of success by using epidermal chalone on the VX2 epidermal tumor although no data had at the time of this writing been published. In other systems, such as for example in the case of malignant leukemic granulocytes, the tumor cells may continue to produce a chalone-like substance capable of inhibiting mitosis in normal granulocytic progenitor cells (434) but they themselves are unable to respond to it (132, 133). Thus, in this instance at least, the chalone system does not appear to function since the tumor cells have become resistant to the inhibitory effect of that substance on the cell division process (99).

The Physiological Basis for Autonomy in Plant Tumors

Insight into the nature of autonomous growth of the plant tumor cell followed an understanding of the factors that regulate normal cell growth and division. Growth in all animals and plants is the result of either the enlargement of cells or the combined processes of cell enlargement and cell division. As has been indicated earlier in this discussion, those fundamental growth processes are controlled in plants by the quantitative interaction of two growth-regulating hormones, the auxins, which are concerned with cell enlargement, and the cytokinins, which act synergistically with the auxins to promote cell growth accompanied by division. Because of the fundamental role that these hormones play in establishing the pattern of synthesis concerned with normal cell growth and division, it appeared likely that they also played a central role in the development of a capacity for autonomous growth of a plant tumor cell.

Normal tobacco pith parenchyma cells have lost, as a result of their maturation and differentiation, the capacity to synthesize these two essential growth-regulating substances. Since the biosynthetic systems required to synthesize these two growth hormones appear to be solidly repressed in normal tobacco pith cells, it was of interest to learn how such cell types would respond when transformed into crown gall tumor cells. The results of such experiments demonstrated that when healing pith parenchyma cells are converted into crown gall tumor cells, non-self-limiting neoplastic overgrowths develop (78) (see Fig. 4). This simple experiment demonstrates, then, that although normal tobacco pith cells did not and could not synthesize physiologically effective amounts of either the cell enlargement hormone or the cell division factor, following their transformation to tumor cells both hormones were produced in greater than regulatory amounts. If that

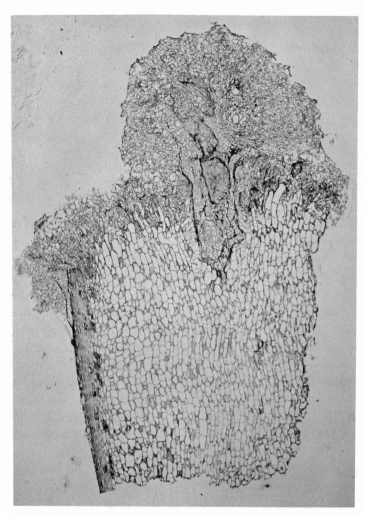

Fig. 4. The transformation and resulting tumor formation of tobacco pith parenchyma cells. Although normal tobacco pith cells do not synthesize auxins or cytokinins, following their transformation to crown gall tumor cells both hormones are synthesized in greater than regulatory amounts. If that were not true, continued growth accompanied by cell division and, hence, tumor formation would not have occurred in this test system (compare with Fig. 3). That the hormones are, in fact, synthesized by crown gall tumor cells was established unequivocally by their isolation and chemical characterization from the tumor tissues. This study demonstrates that a selective and persistent derepression of the host cell genome occurs as a result of the transformation process.

were not true, continued growth accompanied by cell division and, hence, tumor formation would not have resulted in the test system used in those experiments.

That these hormones are actually synthesized by crown gall tumor cells was demonstrated unequivocally by isolating and characterizing chemically those substances. The main cell enlargement hormone was found, as might be expected, to be indole-3-acetic acid while the cell division triggering factor was found to be a new type of compound which has now been partially characterized chemically (569, 572). This interesting substance contains nicotinamide, a glucose sugar moiety, sulfur in the form of sulfate or sulfonate, and one or more methyl groups as well as a straight chain fatty acid(s). This key metabolite, which is continually synthesized by the tumor cells, plays a central role in the development of a capacity for autonomous growth of plant tumor cells, since it keeps such cells dividing persistently.

It is clear from these studies, then, that an essential difference between a normal tobacco pith cell and a crown gall tumor cell is concerned at a physiological level with the permanent activation of two growth substance-synthesizing systems the products of which are concerned specifically with cell growth and division. The continued production in greater than regulatory amounts of these two essential growth-regulating substances could account for the continued unregulated and autonomous proliferation of the crown gall tumor cell. Subsequent studies showed, however, that additional metabolic systems are persistently activated following the transformation of a normal cell into a crown gall tumor cell.

The transformation of a normal plant cell into a fully autonomous crown gall tumor cell is not a one-step process but takes place gradually and progressively over a 3- to 4-day period (Fig. 5). When, for example, the tumor-inducing principle associated with this disease acts on plant cells in an area of irritation for only 34 to 36 hours, very slowly growing tumors develop. A 50-hour exposure of plant cells to the action of that principle results in tumors that grow at a moderately fast rate, while tumors initiated in a 72- to 96-hour period grow very rapidly and the cells of such tumors are fully autonomous (80). The degree of neoplastic change achieved appears to reflect the stage in the normal wound healing cycle in which the cellular transformation occurs (83). It is just before or during the earliest stages of

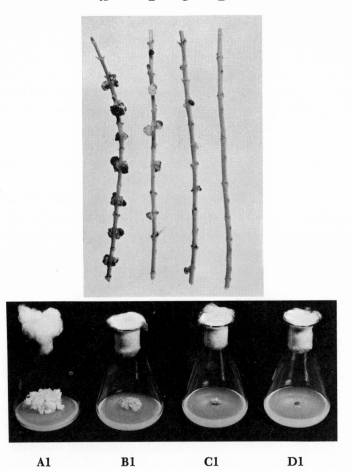

Fig. 5. Tumor progression in the crown gall disease of *Vinca rosea*. *Upper row:* The transformation process was allowed to proceed for **A,** 72 hrs; **B,** 60 hrs; **C,** 34 hrs; **D,** 24 hrs, before it was terminated by means of a thermal treatment. Note no tumors are initiated in 24 hrs. Very small slowly growing tumors are initiated in 34 hrs, moderately fast growing tumors in 60 hrs, while those initiated in 72 or more hrs grow rapidly.

Lower row: **A1,** Sterile tissue isolated from tumors similar to those shown in **A** (above) and planted on White's basic culture medium. **B1,** Tissue isolated from tumors pictured in **B. C1,** Tissue isolated from tumors in **C** (above). **D1,** Normal *Vinca rosea* tissue of the type from which the tumor tissues were derived. The tumor tissues retain indefinitely their characteristic growth patterns on White's basic culture medium. This, then, is an interesting example of tumor progression in which three different grades of neoplastic change can be obtained at will.

active cell division in the healing cycle that normal cells are transformed into tumor cells of the most rapidly growing type (76). Sterile tissues isolated from the three types of tumors described above and planted on a simple basic culture medium composed of mineral salts, sucrose, and three vitamins retain indefinitely in culture their characteristic growth patterns. This, then, represents an interesting example of tumor progression in which different grades of neoplastic change can be obtained at will.

Since these tumor cells retained indefinitely in culture their characteristic growth patterns, they were admirably suited and were used for a study of the factors required for rapid autonomous growth (80). In those studies the rapidly growing fully autonomous tumor cells were used as the standard. Such cell types can synthesize in optimal or near optimal amounts all of the growth factors needed for their continued rapid growth from the mineral salts, sucrose, and three vitamins present in the basic culture medium. The moderately fast growing tumor cell transformed in a 50-hour period required that the basic medium be supplemented with glutamine, myo-inositol, and the cell enlargement hormone auxin to achieve a growth rate equal to that of the fully transformed tumor cell grown on the unsupplemented medium. These were the minimal requirements to achieve that level of growth. That these were the actual requirements was demonstrated experimentally (86, 570). The very slowly growing tumor cells transformed in a 34- to 36-hour period required, in addition to the three compounds described above, asparagine as well as a purine and pyrimidine, the latter requirements being satisfied by guanylic and cytidylic acids, to achieve rapid growth (see Fig. 6). It is clear from such experiments that as the crown gall tumor cell becomes more autonomous, its requirements for rapid growth in terms of exogenously supplied growth factors become less exacting.

Normal cells of the type from which the tumor cells were derived do not grow at all on the basic culture medium. Thus, although the difference between the three types of tumor cells is a quantitative difference since all three grow continuously although at different rates on the basic culture medium, the difference between the tumor cells and the normal cells is qualitative. The exogenous requirements for the rapid growth of normal cells were found to be exactly the same as those required for the rapid growth of the most slowly growing type

Rapidly growing fully altered tumor cells planted on	Moderately fast growing tumor cells planted on	Slowly growing tumor cells planted on	Normal cells planted on
Basic Medium	Basic Medium	Basic Medium	Basic Medium
	Basic Medium + glutamine, inositol, naphthaleneacetic acid	Basic Medium + glutamine, asparagine, inositol, cytidylic & guanylic acids, naphthaleneacetic acid	Basic Medium + glutamine, asparagine, inositol, cytidylic & guanylic acids, 6-furfurylaminopurine, naphthaleneacetic acid

Fig. 6. Relative rates of growth of three tumors that show different degrees of neoplastic change, planted on White's basic culture medium. (*Left*), Fully autonomous tumor cells transformed in a 72-hr period. (*Upper left*), Moderately fast growing tumor cells transformed in a 60-hr period. (*Upper center*), Very slowly growing tumor cells transformed in a 34-hr period. (*Upper right*), Normal cells of the type from which the tumor cells were derived.

Lower pictures and legends show minimal nutritional requirements needed by the three types of tissues to achieve a growth rate comparable to that of the fully autonomous tumor cells shown at left of picture.

of tumor cells with one exception. The normal cells, unlike the tumor cells, possess an absolute exogenous requirement for a cytokinin, the hormone that triggers cell division. All three types of tumor cells have acquired, as a result of their transformation, a capacity to synthesize that hormone. This, then, represents a fundamental difference between a normal cell and a crown gall tumor cell since it is that newly synthesized metabolite that keeps the tumor cells dividing persistently.

Results of experiments such as those described above give a great deal of information concerning the workings of the crown gall tumor system. They indicate, first of all, that as a result of the transition from a normal cell to a fully autonomous rapidly growing tumor cell, a series of quite distinct but well-defined biosynthetic systems, which represent the entire area of metabolism concerned with cell growth and division, become progressively and persistently activated. The degree of activation of those systems determines, moreover, the rate at which the crown gall tumor cell grows.

It is also clear from those studies that autonomy, in this instance, finds its explanation in terms of cellular nutrition. The tumor cells have acquired, as a result of the cellular transformation, a capacity to synthesize all of the essential metabolites that their normal counterparts require but cannot make for cell growth and division.

Finally, those studies demonstrate that as a result of the transition from a normal cell to a fully autonomous tumor cell, a profound and persistent reorientation in the pattern of synthesis occurs. This switch in the pattern of metabolism from that found in a normal resting cell to that present in a persistently dividing cell is triggered by irritation accompanying a wound. That pattern is fixed in the crown gall tumor cell by the tumor-inducing principle responsible for the transformation of normal cell to tumor cell. It is maintained in the plant tumor cell because the two hormones that regulate cell growth and division are continually synthesized by such cell types. The other essential metabolites shown to be produced by tumor cells are required for the synthesis of the nucleic acids, the mitotic and enzymatic proteins and, in the case of inositol, the membrane systems of the cell. These metabolites are essential to permit the pattern of synthesis concerned with cell growth and division to be expressed.

The concept of growth autonomy presented above finds additional support in other directions. It has been possible to reproduce under defined experimental conditions and with the use of normal cell types as the experimental test object not only the morphological growth patterns (slow and rapid disorganized growth, teratoma-like structures) but also the histological (hypertrophy and hyperplasia leading to disorganization and loss of function) as well as the cytological (polyploidy, multinucleate giant cells, etc.) abnormalities that characterize the tumorous state in crown gall (79). This was accomplished by varying the proportions of the cell enlargement hormone, auxin, and the hormone limiting for cell division in an otherwise suitable culture medium. These artificially stimulated normal cells, in contrast to the tumor cells, are self-limiting growths and when the externally applied stimuli are removed growth promptly stops. The fact that such artificially stimulated normal cells commonly show histological and cytological characteristics of true tumor cells but are themselves self-limiting growths indicates that the observed cellular abnormalities are the result rather than the cause of the tumorous state.

It is interesting to note that the development of a capacity for autonomous growth in cells of two other non-self-limiting tumorous diseases of plants, one of which is caused by a virus and the other of which has a genetic basis and requires only nonspecific irritation to initiate tumorous overgrowths, has a physiological basis that is very similar to that described for the crown gall disease (84). These findings indicate that three different and quite distinct proximate causes are capable of redirecting cellular metabolism and accomplishing the same end result largely through a persistent activation of biosynthetic systems that are concerned with cell growth and division.

Evidence for an Extensive Activation of Biosynthetic Systems in Tumor Cells

Plant Tumors

In the crown gall disease such an activation appears to be extensive and the tumor cells may synthesize, in addition to metabolites required specifically for cell growth and division, other substances that their normal counterparts either do not synthesize at all or produce only in limited amounts. An example of this is the new amino acid lysopine (N-αpropionyl-L-lysine) which was first isolated by Lioret (311) in alcohol extracts from crown gall tumor tissue cultures of four different plant species (52). This compound was not initially reported to be present in normal tissues. However, Seitz and Hochster (450) found it to be produced in small amounts by normal tobacco and tomato plants. The tumor tissue from those plant species contained about twenty-four times as much lysopine as did corresponding normal tissues.

More interesting is the finding that the amino acid octopine (N-carboxyethylarginine) is also synthesized in large quantities by crown gall tumor tissues of many different kinds (353, 354). This compound, which was first isolated from octopus muscle, has not, as yet, been found in any normal plant tissue despite an intensive search. The latter example particularly serves to illustrate that as a result of a derepression of the cellular genome following the transformation process, a new compound, which had previously been isolated only from the octopus and other lower animal forms, is produced by tumor tissues of higher plant species. The potentialities for the synthesis of that amino acid were apparently carried through evolutionary development in the genome of many different plant species but only following the cellular transformation were those potentialities expressed.

Another example of an interesting metabolite newly synthesized by crown gall tumor cells and resulting from a persistent activation of a biosynthetic system is that concerned with the production of the cell division-triggering hormone, cytokinin. That compound was found to be a nicotinamide derivative and thus represented a very different class of compounds from the 6-substituted purines which had been known for more than a decade to promote cell division in higher plant species. It appeared possible, therefore, that the synthesis of the new cytokinin found in the tumor tissues resulted from the presence of new genetic information that had been introduced into the cells at the time of their transformation. If that were true, then one would not expect to find a similar type of compound to be present in normal cells that had been stimulated to rapid growth with kinetin (6-furfurylaminopurine) in an otherwise suitable culture medium. It was found, however, that normal cells grown under those conditions synthesized a cell division-promoting factor that was very similar if not identical in its physical, chemical, and biological properties to the cell division factor synthesized by the tumor cells in the absence of an exogenous source of kinetin or other 6-substituted purine (572).

These studies suggest, therefore, that kinetin serves merely to induce the synthesis by normal cell types of a cell division-promoting substance and it is that substance rather than the 6-substituted purines that is directly involved in promoting cell division. Thus, the biosynthetic system responsible for the synthesis of the naturally occurring cell division factor may be persistently activated as a result of the cellular transformation or it may be temporarily activated by kinetin or other 6-substituted purines.

Animal Cells

That an activation of biosynthetic systems leading to the production of new substances occurs in animal tumor cells was clearly recognized shortly after the turn of the present century. Peyton Rous and his associates (429) demonstrated that a cell-free extract of an osteochondrosarcoma of fowl could transform connective tissue in voluntary muscle into osteochondrosarcomas, the cells of which synthesize large amounts of cartilage elements. The implication of this finding was not lost to these investigators for they stated: "It is very remarkable that such an agent should bring about a differentiation ordinarily foreign to the tissue." An interesting recent example of this type is the report of the production of an ACTH-like substance by a primary carcinoma of the lung (340). Another example involves the secretion of gonadotropin from a bronchogenic carcinoma (176). Other examples include a primary cancer of the kidney that secretes parathyroid hormone and a cancer of the bronchus that was reported to synthesize corticotropin, an anterior pituitary hormone.

Of particular interest in this regard are the studies of Abelev et al. (1) who have found that liver tumor cells contain an antigen which is identical to one present in embryonic tissue but is not found in normal adult liver. This suggests that genetic information which was expressed in the embryo and subsequently repressed following differentiation was again expressed in the liver tumor. Results that can be interpreted similarly were reported by Gold and Freedman (205) who worked with a human gastrointestinal tumor.

In addition to the synthesis by tumor cells of substances that are not known to be produced by their normal counterparts, there are numerous examples of tumors that secrete excessive amounts of biologically important substances. This is particularly well illustrated in the hormone-secreting endocrine tumors where, for example, islet cell carcinomas of the pancreas may produce huge amounts of insulin even when very small in size. Similarly, pituitary tumors may synthesize large quantities of trophic hormones which may result in gigantism or acromegaly from growth hormone excess and in Cushing's syndrome from an excess of ACTH, while thyroid carcinomas may give rise to extreme hyperthyroidism. Myelomas can, moreover, produce large amounts of γ-globulins without apparently any initiating antigenic factor (395). These, then, are prime examples in the plant and animal fields of altered control mechanisms which reflect a persistent activation of biosynthetic systems other than those concerned specifically with cell growth and division.

Plant Tumors as a Model for
Understanding Autonomous Growth

Can the concepts that have been developed to explain autonomous growth of plant tumor cells be made to serve as a model for the tumor problem generally? Several points of interest emerge from an analysis of plant tumor systems. It appears, first of all, that despite different and quite distinct initiating causes in the three non-self-limiting tumorous diseases described above—Black's wound tumor disease which is caused by an RNA virus, the crown gall disease initiated by a tumor-inducing principle, and the tumor-forming hybrids which require only nonspecific irritation—the underlying physiological and biochemical basis for autonomous growth is very similar in all. In these instances the tumor cells have acquired as a result of their transformation the capacity to synthesize persistently all of the metabolites that their normal counterparts require but cannot make for continued cell growth and division. These studies also show, and this will be documented in Chapter VI, that the normal and tumor cell nuclei are genetically equivalent in two and possibly in the third of these neoplastic diseases. Thus in these three instances the heritable cellular changes that lead to autonomous growth appear to be of an epigenetic type involving changes in the *expression* of the genetic potentialities present in a cell rather than changes in the integrity of the genetic information involving a loss or permanent rearrangement of the genetic information that is normally present in a cell.

In all of these instances, then, the heritable cellular changes leading to the development of a capacity for autonomous growth appear to result from a persistent activation of certain normally repressed biosynthetic systems. This leads to the continued synthesis by the tumor cells of all of the essential metabolites required for continued cell growth and division. Even in the case of Black's wound tumor disease where enough genetic information in the form of viral RNA is introduced into a cell at the time of transformation to code for more than twenty-five new proteins, the mechanism underlying tumorous growth appears basically to be one involving an activation of repressed biosynthetic systems. It seems most unlikely that this new information codes for the synthesis of the two hormones and the other metabolites that are normally required for the cell division process in plants. In the crown gall disease this persistent activation appears to be dependent, in part at least, on changes in the properties of the membrane systems that accompany the neoplastic transformation.

While differences in particulars doubtless exist, there nevertheless appears to be little in the literature that argues strongly against a similar mechanism involving a persistent activation of certain normally repressed biosynthetic systems as the underlying basis of the tumorous state in animal systems. We shall examine in the next chapter alternative types of heritable changes in cells and attempt to determine whether any of these offer a more satisfactory explanation for the origin of a tumor cell. Before getting into a discussion of that aspect of the problem, one additional point requires consideration.

The Surface Properties of Normal and Tumor Cells

Animal Cells

In addition to the loss or partial loss of the mechanisms that normally control cell growth and division, a second process, which is particularly pertinent to the animal tumor field, involves the loss or partial loss by malignant cells of normal contact relations. It is a common observation that as cells become malignant they escape from normal contact relations. This, in turn, leads to a capacity of such cells to infiltrate normal tissues and to detach from a mass of cells and metastasize to distant sites. Aside from leukocytes, macrophages, etc., cells in an adult animal do not normally migrate and invade normal tissues. Morphogenetic cell movements are, on the other hand, very important in normal embryonic development, as was conclusively demonstrated by Holtfreter (243). It is now well known that shifting patterns of adhesiveness are essential in controlling cell movements, in the innervation of organs, and in the blocking out of organs and tissues, as well as in the process of wound healing. Abercrombie, Ambrose, and their co-workers have examined cells *in vitro* and have attempted to quantify certain of the observed effects (3).

Normal fibroblast or epithelial cells in culture are known to migrate actively on a glass or plasma surface. The membranes of such cells are in continuous activity. Ruffles, which may be quite large extending 5 μ or more in height, seem to form continuously across the surface of a cell although those at the leading edge appear to be dominant. Isolated fibroblasts and epithelial cells migrate across glass by membrane undulation which gives rise to intermittent contact with the surface. The sequence of events leading to the formation of ruffled membranes is still obscure although Abercrombie and Heaysman (4) have clearly established that their formation is inhibited by contact with another cell. When the ruffled membrane of a migrating fibroblast comes in contact with that of another fibroblast the membranes become paralyzed, the two cells adhere to one another and cell movement comes to a halt. Since the movement of normal fibroblasts is controlled by contact with other similar cells they tend to line up in parallel fashion in monolayer culture and, if movement occurs, to migrate as a parallel group of cells.

Carcinoma or sarcoma cells, when grown in culture, commonly behave quite differently from their normal counterparts. The tumor cells often assume a rounded form but instead of showing one dominant ruffled membrane they produce a number of pseudopodia, each of which has a ruffled membrane. The movement of the tumor cells is therefore less coordinated although the mechanism of movement appears to be similar to that found in the normal cells. When the ruffled membrane of a tumor cell comes in contact with a normal cell it is not paralyzed and the former moves actively across the normal cell, treating it much as it treats a solid substrate. For this reason in monolayer culture the tumor cells pile up on top of each other in random fashion and the characteristic alignment found in cultured normal cells is not observed (see Fig. 14). This finding has been widely used to distinguish normal cells from tumor cells in culture. A good correlation has been found to exist, moreover, between the ability of a tumor to invade and metastasize in a host and the loss of contact inhibition of such cells when grown in monolayer culture (19).

The possible relationship between contact inhibition and cell division is interesting because of the association of increased cell division within malignant cell populations with a deficiency of contact inhibition. Normal fibroblasts in division also round up and show a deficiency in contact inhibition. It is conceivable that in both normal and tumor cells the division mechanism is affected by the surface change. It is, nevertheless, evident that mitotic rates can increase without appreciably diminishing contact inhibition.

While morphological conversions appear to be characteristic of neoplastic cells of many types, there are exceptions. Sanford and collaborators (443), for example, carried out an extensive series of experiments with the Rous sarcoma virus in cultures of chick cells and found that, although multiplication of the virus and the production of tumors were demonstrable with these cell populations, the characteristic morphological conversions did not occur. Similarly, Prince (407) did not observe significant morphological changes in cultures of chick and turkey fibroblasts infected with Rous virus although the cells were demonstrably virus-producers. In this instance the discrepancy was eventually explained by adding tryptose phosphate broth to the culture medium, indicating the importance of environmental factors for the expression of the morphological changes.

Defendi and associates (146), in a paper entitled " 'Morphologically normal' hamster cells with malignant properties," have pointed out that loss of contact inhibition is not a necessary factor for the acquisition of transplantability. It should also be noted in this connection (487) that early BHK21 hamster cells, which do not possess the high transplantability of a spontaneous variant, have the same unrestricted growth potential in culture. It has also been found that although transformed cells may not show contact inhibition with other transformed cells of the same type, cells transformed by the polyoma virus (488), by methylcholanthrene (51), by X-irradiation (65), and "spontaneously" (33) are contact-inhibited by normal cells. Borek and Sachs (65) have found, moreover, that cells transformed by one carcinogen may be contact-inhibited by cells transformed by another carcinogen. These workers conclude from their studies that normal cells are contact-inhibited by the same or by a different cell type while transformed cells are inhibited only by a different cell type. Easty (165) indicates that certain carcinomas exhibit considerable mutual contact inhibition in monolayer culture but nevertheless possess a capacity to invade *in vivo*.

The recent experiments of Holley and Kiernan (241) suggest that the concept of contact inhibition in normal cells and the loss thereof by many tumor cell types may require re-evaluation. These investigators demonstrated that the final density to which 3T3 cells grow in culture is simply a function of the concentration of serum in the nutrient medium. The final cell count varied directly with serum concentration, and while 10% calf serum produced a confluent monolayer, greater serum concentrations produced final cell densities far in excess of that found in one monolayer. Polyoma-transformed 3T3 cells were found to have a decreased requirement for the serum factor(s) and always grew to a greater final density than did the nontransformed 3T3 cells at a given serum concentration. The fact that the nontransformed 3T3 cells yielded a monolayer in a 10% calf-serum-containing medium while polyoma-transformed 3T3 cells grew in excess of a monolayer was erroneously interpreted to mean that the untransformed 3T3 cells possessed a "contact inhibition" of growth while the transformants did not. When serum concentrations greater than 10% were used both 3T3 cells and transformed 3T3 cells grew beyond a monolayer, thus demonstrating that the phenomenon of contact inhibition does not exist, at least not in this system.

The changes in behavior of a malignant cell appear, nevertheless, to be related to changes in the adhesiveness of the cell surface. Since the initial observations of Coman in 1944 it has been recognized that animal cancer cells are more easily separated from each other than are cells of benign tumors or of corresponding normal tissues (126). It was found that the force needed to separate normal cells was approximately twice that required to separate carcinoma cells. Coman (128) suggested on the basis of his studies that the reduced adhesiveness found in cancer cells constituted a physical basis of malignancy and indicated that it might explain both invasion and metastases. He suggested further that the reduced calcium content of cancer cells was correlated with diminished adhesive properties of the cell surface. Some years later Coman (127) reported that within an hour or so after application of the carcinogenic hydrocarbon 7,12-dimethylbenzanthrene to the ear of a rabbit, membranes of the exposed cells showed lowered adhesiveness. This was not found to be true when noncarcinogenic anthracene was similarly applied.

A change in adhesiveness in a cell surface can arise either from a decrease in attractive forces between surfaces or an increase in repulsive forces. Electrophoretic studies, which measure the charge per unit area on the cell surface that is almost independent of cell size, have shown that the net negative surface charge was higher on the surface of tumor cells than on comparable normal cell types in a number of different and quite distinct systems studied (19). There appears, moreover, to be increasing evidence that tumor progression leading to greater malignancy is associated with increasing surface charge density.

The chemical nature of the material on the cell surface that is responsible for the surface charge has been investigated. Such studies were possible because of the finding that phospholipids, an important constituent of cell membranes, have a certain affinity for calcium ions while the sialic-acid-containing component does not and the latter is specifically degraded by the enzyme neuraminidase. It is thus quite possible to distinguish between sialic acid and phospholipid on the cell surface by treatment with either neuraminidase or calcium ions. It has been found, for example, that in mature human red cells 90% of the surface charge per unit area may be removed by treatment with the enzyme neuraminidase, thus indicating that most of the surface charge in that cell type is due to the carboxyl groups of the sialic acid. The surfaces of human erythrocytes have little or no affinity for calcium ions (19).

By applying this method to cloned hamster cells transformed by the polyoma virus and to cloned normal counterparts it was possible to show, first of all, that the transformed cells showed a greater electrophoretic mobility than did the normal cell types. Treatment of both cell types with calcium ions reduced the mobility of the tumor cells somewhat but differences could still be observed. When, on the other hand, both cell types were treated with neuraminidase, mobility in an electrophoretic field was found to be identical in the transformed and normal cells. This finding suggests that a sialic-acid-containing component is largely responsible for the surface charge on the polyoma-transformed tumor cells. Similar results were obtained when the EL-4 leukemia cells were used as the experimental test object. With Ehrlich ascites tumor cells, on the other hand, exposed phospholipid groups were also found to be present (19).

The sialic acid component has been found to be a sialomucopeptide containing sialic acid as a terminal group and N-acetylgalactosamine. The sugar appears to be linked to the peptide by glutamic acid while the peptide has an amino acid composition that is rather similar to collagen (19).

It is interesting to note that Landschütz ascites tumor cells were rendered immunogenic in A2G mice by prior *in vitro* treatment with neuraminidase (135). This led to the subsequent immunity to inoculation with the untreated tumor. It was concluded from that study that the surface antigens of the ascites tumor cells are masked by the sialic acid moiety of the sialomucopeptides at the surface of the tumor cells. These results suggest that the free carboxyl groups of the sialic acid, by conferring a high negative charge to the cell periphery, inhibit the approach of lymphoid cells and thus inhibit antigen detection.

Certain normal cells such as the lymphocytes and macrophages, which, like malignant cells, show low adhesiveness, are able to invade extensively normal tissues but do not possess the property of malignancy. This can doubtless be explained by the fact that the cellular mechanisms that control mitosis and cell division in the mature normal cell types are precisely regulated and hence the essentially uncontrolled cell division required for neoplastic growth does not occur. Thus, two processes are crucially involved in the cancerous transformation. Cells must lose, partially or completely, their growth control mechanisms and their normal surface properties.

One further point, dealing with differences in intercellular communication, should be considered. Penn (392) and Loewenstein and Kanno (320) have found that in normal liver cells the junctional membrane surfaces are freely permeable to small ions and possibly to large ions and molecules. In tumorous growths of the liver, on the other hand, the junctional membranes, if they exist at all in a functional state, are relatively impermeable even to the smaller ions. In this respect the tumor cells are similar in behavior to normal cells after their junctional membranes have been blocked with uncoupling agents (369). Thus, while there appears to be ample room for the exchange of substances between adjoining normal cells, there is virtually none in the case of the tumor cells studied.

Intercellular communication was also examined in regenerating rat liver and in wounded urodele skin, which are two tissues that grow rapidly but normally (321). In both of these instances cellular communication was generally found to be good in their respective normal intact states. Upon wounding of urodele skin the normally permeable junctional membranes sealed themselves off, thus sealing the interior of the cell from the exterior. When, during wound closure, the cells of two opposing borders made contact, communication between them was restored within thirty minutes. This is in striking contrast to the lack of cellular communication found in certain cells of cancerous origin. Yet, as Loewenstein and Kanno (320) point out, the place within the causal chain of cancer occupied by junctional communication is not at all clear at present because good electrical communication has recently been shown to exist between certain mouse and hamster fibroblasts transformed by oncogenic viruses.

Finally, another property of malignant animal cells is their increased permeability to macromolecules and this is almost certainly due to changes in the cell surface (109a).

Plant Cells

The importance of the surface properties of cells in the establishment of the malignant state in animals appears now to be well founded. Profound changes that play a central role in the development of a capacity for autonomous growth also occur in the properties of the membrane systems of the plant tumor cell. It has been found that during the transition from a normal cell to a fully autonomous rapidly growing crown gall tumor cell, gradual and progressive increases in the permeability of the cell membranes occur not only for inorganic ions but for certain organic solutes as well (571). Those studies have shown, moreover, that five and in part six of the seven essential biosynthetic systems found to be persistently activated in the plant tumor cell can be rendered functional in normal cell types by specific ions. Only the biosynthetic system concerned with the synthesis of the cell division-promoting hormone, cytokinin, cannot as yet be accounted for on that basis.

It has thus been possible to replace many of the exogenously required organic metabolites needed for continued rapid cell growth and division in normal cell types simply by raising the concentration of certain ions in the basic culture medium. The fully autonomous tumor cell takes up ions very efficiently from dilute salt solutions; the normal cells do not. This, then, represents a fundamental difference between the fully autonomous tumor cell and its normal counterpart since a large segment of metabolism concerned specifically with cell growth and division is rendered fully functional by specific ions.

Since the properties of membrane systems of both animal and plant tumor cells play a fundamental role in determining the activities of those cells, it would appear of prime importance to learn whether or not membrane changes such as those found in tumor cells can be perpetuated hereditarily without corresponding changes in the genotype of a cell. Rubin (432) has considered this question and suggests that the phenomenon that Sonneborn (467) has named cytotaxis and which involves the ordering and arranging of new cell structure under the influence of pre-existing cell structure in the absence of genic change, may be applicable to membranes. If that is true then Willmer's (562) suggestion that some of the most potent carcinogens such as methylcholanthrene, the benzpyrenes, and the dibenzanthracenes are likely, because of their solubility properties, to localize preferentially in the membranes and exert their primary carcinogenic effect there would be understandable.

It has been difficult in the past to explain how alterations in membrane properties caused by the carcinogenic hydrocarbons could be perpetuated in progeny cells in the absence of the original carcinogen itself. Sonneborn and his co-workers (46) have shown, however, that by modifying the normal pattern of structure in *Paramecium* in various ways to yield two or more mouths and gullets in various positions or by modifying the pattern of the cortex by grafting methods, such modifications are inherited by the progeny at successive cell divisions and even through sexual reproduction. Studies on what amounted to nuclear transplantations in both directions between the modified and normal cells as well as standard breeding analysis showed that these differences were not due either to differences in the genes present or to gene activity. They were due only to differences in the initial cell structure and organization.

It must therefore be concluded from these studies that the higher levels of organization of cortical units at the surface of the organism are determined by the arrangement of pre-existing units. It is a type of heritable change and a form of cellular differentiation that is quite distinct in principle from that concerned either with somatic mutation at the nuclear gene level or with variable gene activity which will be considered in a following chapter. It would appear most important for metazoan biologists to find appropriate means to determine whether or not membrane changes can be perpetuated hereditarily without genic changes. If they can, it would be important to learn how the patterns can be modified hereditarily and what role such modifications play in differentiation and malignancy (432).

CHAPTER IV

On the Nature of
the Heritable Cellular Change

Somatic Mutation

One of the most firmly held beliefs in the field of oncology is that once a cell has been converted to the malignant state the change is permanent and irreversible. This concept of irreversibility has completely dominated the thinking of most cancer biologists and many have over the years favored the theory of somatic cell mutation to account for the apparent irreversibility of the cancerous state. Credit for this theory as it applies to the tumor problem is generally given to Boveri (72) who in 1914 reported that malignant cells, when examined microscopically, almost always contain a grossly abnormal complement of chromosomes; he concluded that this abnormal condition was the cause of the malignant state. The theory of somatic mutation is favored by many today although the definitions of somatic cell mutation often used are so vague as to be essentially useless as a guide for experimentation. In a recently published book on the genesis and biology of cancer (272) the author perhaps best sums up the type of thinking that has led to the acceptance by many of the mutation theory of cancer. He states:

The premises justifying the conclusion that mutation takes place begins with dicta on biological behaviour that have been accepted for a century or more. If "all cells come from pre-existing cells," as proclaimed by Virchow in 1855; and "all cells come from genetically similar parent cells," as asserted by Thiersch 10 years later; and cancer cells originate from normal body cells, then somewhere along the line of change from normalcy to malignancy there must be one or more mutations.

This type of reasoning, which is not at all uncommon, precludes the existence of heritable cellular changes other than those caused by mutation.

If the term somatic mutation is used, as it is often used, to describe the obvious fact that profound and heritable changes occur during the transition from a normal cell to a tumor cell, then it is pretentious as a descriptive term and carries with it a connotation that tends to stifle precision of thought. If, on the other hand, by somatic mutation is meant that there is a permanent change in the integrity of the genetic information that is normally present in the nucleus of a cell, then the term designates a hypothesis that remains untestable by the classical Mendelian methods because tumor cells propagate themselves only vegetatively. The newer methods of somatic cell hybridization do, however, shed light on this question and these will be considered later in this discussion.

Evidence in Support of Somatic Mutation

What, then, is the evidence to support the somatic mutation theory of cancer? The proponents of this theory advance essentially four main types of arguments in its support. The first of these is the great frequency with which chromosomal abnormalities are associated with the malignant state, the second concerns itself with the presumed correlation that exists between mutagenic and carcinogenic agents, the third is based on the finding that deletion of cellular constituents may often accompany the tumorous state, while the fourth postulates the addition and integration of new genetic information into the genome of a cell.

Chromosomal Anomalies. The idea that abnormal complements of chromosomes may be etiologically involved in malignant growth stems from the early studies of Klebs who in 1889 reported that some cancer cells had many chromosomes while others had few. This work was followed by the detailed investigations of Hansemann who, over a period of sixteen years, made detailed studies of chromosomal and mitotic abnormalities in human tumors and suggested that the observed anomalies might be causally related to the tumorous state. This suggestion was put into definitive form by Boveri (72) who, in his book *The Origin of Malignant Tumors*, wrote: "The essence of my theory, is not abnormal mitosis, but in general, a definite *abnormal chromosome-complex.*" With the development of new cytological techniques much information about the behavior of chromosomes in normal as well as in tumor cells has become available in the past two decades. Through the use of these methods, chromosomal anomalies of many different kinds have been observed in many different tumors of animals and man. The high incidence with which such anomalies are found would appear, moreover, to provide evidence in favor of the Boveri theory. Yet, with very few exceptions (382, 383, 499, 536), which are perhaps best exemplified by chronic myelocytic leukemia in humans, the observed chromosomal anomalies commonly found in cancer cells show no consistent pattern.

It is not uncommon, moreover, to find a variety of karyotypes within any given tumor. A sequence of stem lines each with its own peculiar karyotype may be observed to follow one another during the progression of a tumor. Levan (302) has suggested that deviations from the original karyotype found in advanced tumors may be regarded as a manifestation of genetic evolution in which the dominating stem line represents those cells which are best adapted to their immediate environment. If and when the environment changes, other stem lines which are better able to adapt to the new conditions become dominant. It would thus appear that the presence of different karyotypes within a tumor would confer a very real selective advantage as far as the growth of the tumor is concerned. This does not necessarily mean, of course, that such karyotypic anomalies are etiologically involved in the basic mechanisms underlying tumorigenesis. They may well be the result rather than the cause of the tumorous state.

In the generality of tumors, then, carcinogenesis does not lead to characteristic karyotypic patterns. A dramatic exception to this, however, is the case of chronic myelocytic leukemia of humans. In this disease an excellent correlation has been found to exist between the presence of an abnormal chromosome in the malignant cells and the disease. The Philadelphia chromosome (Ph^1), which is one of the G group of chromosomes, has lost approximately one-half of the long arm and is believed to be a highly specific morphological marker for chronic myelocytic leukemia. It is not at present known whether the chromosome fragment has been deleted from the cell or whether it has been translocated to another chromosome within the karyotype. It has been found (516), moreover, that in those instances in which the Ph[1] chromosome is entirely absent from the cell, life expectancy is only 18 months as compared with 45 months when the Ph[1] chromosome is present. This, then, would appear to be a classical example of somatic cell mutation in which the loss of a chromosome segment or, in more extreme cases, of the entire chromosome, is involved. In either case it may be postulated that the missing component harbors the nuclear genes concerned with the regulation of growth.

Such a concept would appear to be strengthened by the finding that advanced tumors of other kinds may show a deficiency of G type chromosomes. It has been found, for example, that certain human cell types transformed *in vitro* by the SV40 virus show a loss of G type chromosomes (577, 364). Very recent studies (399, 409a) on the normalization of cells transformed by DNA-containing viruses raise serious questions concerning the significance of chromosome deletion as the mechanism underlying tumorigenesis in these systems.

Even in the case of chronic myelocytic leukemia the correlation between the presence of the Ph[1] chromosome and the disease appears not to be a perfect one. In different investigations the frequency of Ph[1]-positive patients has varied from 66% to 100%. The tendency has been to interpret the negative findings as being attributable to difficulties either with the cytological technique or in the diagnosis of the disease. Nevertheless, because of these exceptions, the etiological relationship between the Ph[1] chromosome and chronic myelocytic leukemia has not been unequivocally established and remains a correlation.

The relation of the Ph[1] chromosome to the disease is interesting from another point of view. It appears that in chronic myelocytic leukemia it is the stem cells found in the bone marrow and perhaps the immature granulocytes in the blood that proliferate in abnormal numbers. The progeny of those cells found in the peripheral blood mature and differentiate during the chronic phase of the disease and do not appear to show a capacity for autonomous growth. Although such mature cells may differ from their normal counterparts in certain respects, e.g., loss or low levels of lysosomal alkaline phosphatase, they do retain many normal functions. It has been reported, moreover, that not only the granulocytic cells but also the erythrocytic and megakaryocytic cells, all of which probably arise from a common precursor, may contain the Ph[1] chromosome, and yet in the latter two instances there commonly is no excessive cell proliferation. If it is true, then, that mature differentiated cells lack a capacity for autonomous proliferation and that cells other than the granulocytes contain the Ph[1] chromosome but do not necessarily replicate autonomously, the conclusion seems unmistakable that the presence of the Ph[1] chromosome in a cell is not in itself sufficient to cause that cell to proliferate in an unrestrained manner.

It is now perfectly clear, moreover, that a significant number of malignant tumors do exist with a predominantly normal diploid karyotype (29, 41, 152, 229, 249, 294, 322). The question has, therefore, been raised (394) as to whether chromosomal anomalies such as aneuploidy and related phenomena are primary causes or secondary effects of the malignant process. Extensive studies in various tissue culture systems have failed for the most part to uncover any correlations between aneuploidy and malignancy (34, 249, 303, 420, 539). In fact, aneuploidy typically occurs very early after cells are placed in culture while malignancy commonly occurs much later or not at all. Thus, aneuploidy in itself is not an adequate indicator of malignancy.

Arguments of the type presented above do not, of course, preclude the possibility that there may be microscopic changes in the genetic material present in a cell and that it is those changes rather than the more crude shifts in karyotype pattern that are involved in establishing the malignant state. A modified mutation theory of cancer based on such small microscopic changes in the genome of a cell has been proposed by Nichols (373). Because of the inadequacies of present methods, it is difficult to put such a theory to experimental test except perhaps in certain exceptional instances, one of which is described below. Albert Levan and his associates have indicated that certain mammalian cells including hamster cells transformed by the Schmidt-Ruppin strain of the Rous sarcoma virus may show an increased incidence of chromosome breakage and this involved specific chromosome types more often than others. These workers (374) feel that these chromosome breaks may be etiologically significant and may act as an indicator system for point mutations. They suggest, further, that such breaks may be similar to those induced by X rays in which the number of breaks reflects the incidence of mutation and mutagenic activity. Thus, according to these investigators, chromosome breakage can provide a common denominator of the three agents that are known to produce cancer: chemicals, X-irradiation, and viruses.

The studies of Macpherson (330) on the reversion of hamster cells transformed by the Schmidt-Ruppin strain of the Rous sarcoma virus bear on this question. These studies, which will be taken up in greater detail in Chapter VI, have demonstrated unequivocally that transformed cell clones give rise to a significant percentage of re-vertants that appear to be normal in every respect. This reversion appears, moreover, to be correlated with the loss or partial loss of the Rous sarcoma virus genome carried by the transformed cells. It would thus appear that the chromosome breakage observed by Levan and his associates in hamster cells transformed by the Schmidt-Ruppin strain of the Rous sarcoma virus cannot be directly concerned with the basic mechanism underlying tumorigenesis in this system. The viral genome itself, rather than mutation resulting from chromosome breaks caused by the virus, appears to determine the fate of the cell.

The question as to whether the presence of an excess of specific chromosomes in a tumor cell might be etiologically involved in tumorigenesis has recently been investigated. It had been observed by Hayflick and Moorhead (233) that cultures of normal human diploid cells stop dividing after some 50 to 60 generations. It has very recently been noted (115) that after about 55 cell generations the E16 chromosome content of the cells drops below the normal diploid level and the cells then stop dividing and die. With cancer cells ob-tained either from primary growths or from established lines main-tained in culture the story is different. These show an E16 excess, in both relative and absolute terms. This, then, represents an interesting correlation which deserves further intensive study. Yet it is not so much a question of an excess of particular chromosomes that is im-portant but rather a question of what, if anything, the genetic informa-tion present in those chromosomes is doing specifically to render the cells neoplastic.

One of the reasons given by those who oppose the mutation theory of cancer is that somatic cell mutation is in itself a relatively rare event and that for a fully autonomous cancer to develop it must be postulated that a number of successive mutations are required. Nord-ling (379), for example, has argued on the basis of the relationship between cancer death and age that seven successive mutations are needed to explain that relationship. In the course of criticism of the mutation hypothesis Hieger (239) also argues that acceptance of that concept requires a series of successive mutations and that if in addition one considers the multicentric origin of many tumors, it reduces the probability of the initiation of a cancer based on the mutation hypothesis practically to zero.

However, arguments such as those presented above omit a number of important considerations. They do not take fully into account the possibility that certain carcinogenic agents (e.g., X-irradiation) may significantly increase mutation rate in certain normal cell types. Nor do they take into consideration the fact that extensive gene damage may occur in essentially nondividing somatic cells of mammals. Curtis (137) has presented evidence to suggest that nondividing mammalian cells accumulate mutations at such a rate that by late middle age "virtually all cells carry many gene mutations." It is interesting to note in this connection that while in mitotically inert tissues mutations build up to a high level, in mitotically active tissues Curtis finds such mutations to be rare. It is, however, in the mitotically active tissues that cancers arise most frequently (99).

It might be noted further, however, that patients with Fanconia's anemia characteristically have aneuploid cells. The incidence of tumors of various kinds in such patients is higher than is found in the general population (194) and such aneuploid cells can be transformed much more readily than normal diploid cells by the SV40 virus (518).

Finally, the arguments that have been advanced against the mutation theory of cancer omit consideration of the possibility that gene damage or failure may be at least partly dependent on inherent gene weaknesses, whatever that may mean at the molecular level; according to Burch (102, 103, 104) the majority of malignancies in such animals as man may, in fact, be of this kind.

Correlations between Mutagenicity and Carcinogenicity. Certain chemical compounds as well as physical agents such as radiation may produce mutations, chromosomal anomalies, and tumors. Those instances in which a correlation has been found to exist between mutagenicity and carcinogenicity have provided a most appealing argument for proponents of the somatic mutation theory of cancer. Yet, Burdette (108), in a comprehensive review of the relationship of mutagens to carcinogens concludes that "Those investigators who have tested a wide range of different compounds have found no parallelism between mutagenicity and carcinogenicity." There is, nevertheless, clearly a degree of overlap of the two properties, while there are, on the other hand, many instances in which the two do not run parallel. It is now known, however, that certain compounds with carcinogenic action have first to be converted into their actual carcinogenic derivatives by special enzymes in the tissues before they are effective. Trainin et al. point out that it is possible that only a small proportion of mutagenic agents would share a common site or sites of action which one would postulate to be involved in the initiation of tumors (522).

Even in the case of ultraviolet and X-irradiation where the parallel between mutagenicity and carcinogenicity appears close, Blum (62) and Brues (96) find mutation to be an inadequate explanation for the origin of tumors. Nevertheless, Berenblum and Trainin (49) have demonstrated that radiation carcinogenesis may occur as a two-stage process. Burch (105, 106, 107) also believes that genetic changes may be among the initial events in radiation-induced leukemogenesis. Ideally, mutagenic and carcinogenic properties of physical or chemical agents should be tested in the same organism. This is often not easily accomplished. However, Smith (462), working with an interspecific hybrid within the genus *Nicotiana* which had a high rate of spontaneous tumor formation after the plants reached the flowering stage, demonstrated that doses of gamma irradiation which caused a noticeable increase in the frequency of somatic mutations of a marker gene failed to increase significantly the rate of tumor formation over that found in unirradiated control plants. Sachs and his collaborators (50, 51, 64) have found, moreover, that up to 2% of normal hamster cells treated with 300 γ of X-irradiation became transformed into tumor cells; as many as 20% may be transformed *in vitro* with carcinogenic hydrocarbons. Such a frequency of transformation is much higher than would be expected for randomly occurring mutations.

There appears, then, to be no unequivocal demonstration of structural gene mutations being etiologically involved in establishing the tumorous state. What about regulatory gene mutations? Here, according to Pitot and Cho (395), there are many, too many in fact, to be credible. In almost every mechanism the neoplastic hepatic cell is defective at the transcriptional or translational level in some way. The perplexing fact, according to Pitot, is that the defects are not consistent, each tumor appearing to have an almost unique set of defects. If gene mutations are involved, then each tumor has its own peculiar set all leading to a unique phenotype, the common denominator of which is uncontrolled growth. While this would appear most improbable it is not impossible, as pointed out by Potter (403). Findings of the type described raise the question as to whether there are, in fact, mechanisms other than gene mutation that can more realistically explain metabolic changes of a heritable type such as those described above. This question will be considered further in Chapter V.

The Deletion Hypotheses. Deletions of cellular constituents and activities, which could be attributable to mutations, have been described as occurring in many different tumors. The Millers in 1947 advanced, on the basis of their studies on azo-dye-induced carcinogenesis of the liver, the theory that carcinogenesis results from "a permanent alteration or loss of proteins essential for the control of growth" (358). This conclusion was based on the finding that livers of rats fed aminoazo dyes contained protein with covalently bonded carcinogen, or one of its products, while there was a complete absence of carcinogen binding to the tumor proteins. This work has been confirmed and extended by Sorof and his associates (470) who found that most of the bound dye was present in an electrophoretically slow-moving class of proteins which were termed the h2 proteins. These workers (471) have shown, moreover, that azo-dye-induced liver tumors contain almost none of this class of proteins in the cytoplasm or in the nucleus. In an extension of the deletion hypothesis to other systems, Miller (357) has shown that the carcinogenic hydrocarbon 3,4-benzpyrene is bound to proteins of mouse skin, while Abell and Heidelberger (2) have found that in skin carcinogenic hydrocarbons bind to h2-like soluble proteins whose concentration is much reduced in epidermoid carcinomas.

In addition to protein binding, certain carcinogens (341, 331) such as N-acetyl aminofluorene and ethionine are bound covalently to liver RNA, while other carcinogenic hydrocarbons bind to mouse skin DNA

(93). These findings tend to carry the deletion hypothesis to the level of the gene and its immediate products. The Millers (359) have recently reviewed the interaction of carcinogenic compounds with macromolecules.

In 1950 Potter (401) modified the original deletion hypothesis and suggested that deletions during carcinogenesis may be associated with enzymes involved in catabolic reactions rather than with anabolic synthesis. This was known as the catabolic deletion hypothesis and evidence supporting that hypothesis was reviewed in detail eight years later (402). However, with careful study of the highly differentiated but transplantable "minimal deviation" hepatomas of the rat it became evident that this type of tumor, at least, did not conform either to the original deletion hypothesis of the Millers or with Potter's version of the catabolic deletion hypothesis. The discovery of the striking biochemical similarity between the "minimal deviation" hepatomas and normal liver cells necessitated a critical re-evaluation not only of the deletion hypothesis but of the Warburg (540) and Greenstein (213) hypotheses as well. Potter has now suggested that the catabolic deletion hypothesis may have little relevance to the neoplastic transformation itself but may find application in the progression of tumors.

In 1964 Potter (403) proposed the feedback deletion hypothesis of carcinogenesis which is, in part at least, an outgrowth of the original deletion hypothesis. This theory was proposed largely in support of the concept that cancer results from one or more genetic alterations. A major point of this hypothesis is an attempted explanation of the several-stage theory of skin carcinogenesis described by Boutwell (67) in which an initial mutational event or events not necessarily affecting mechanisms of cell replication is postulated. This is followed by additional mutational events in which each new mutation occurs in a previously mutated cell leading ultimately to the growth and progression of a tumor. Potter interprets the data obtained with the use of "minimal deviation" hepatomas, which show marked divergences one from the other, as resulting from both "essential" and "nonessential" mutations. The essential mutations, according to this interpretation, are those directly involved in mitoses and cell division. Roth (419) has suggested that fewer mutations may be involved and that mutation of a gene related to the histone control of gene expression may be all that is required.

Somatic Cell Hybridization as a Test for the Deletion Hypotheses.
The deletion hypothesis in its various forms has now been put to
experimental test with the use of the recently introduced methods of
somatic cell hybridization. Somatic cell hybridization was discovered
by Barski and his associates in 1960 (36, 37). These investigators
found that when two mouse cell lines of different karyotype are grown
together in culture, a new hybrid cell type appears which is characterized by the presence of the chromosomes of the parental lines. Thus,
somatic cell hybridization provides a powerful new tool for studies
in somatic cell genetics. The results of numerous studies (32, 35, 36,
37, 143, 145, 199, 444, 453, 469) have now been reported in which
tumor cells of various types have been hybridized with normal cells
or with very low tumor-producing cell lines and without exception
the resulting hybrids have retained the tumorous properties when
implanted into suitable hosts. This fact, at least for the systems
studied, is incompatible with deletion hypotheses which postulate that
the cancerous state results from the loss of some essential protein.

The results of hybridization studies do not, however, preclude the
rather remote possibility that an operator locus, if, in fact, such exists
in cells of higher animals, may have been deleted from tumor cells.
The operator locus is believed in bacteria to interact directly with a
specific repressor, thus controlling the function of an adjacent operon.
If an operator is absent, the corresponding repressor cannot inhibit
the synthesis of the specific mRNA and, hence, there is constitutive
synthesis of the corresponding protein. Since the operator in the
bacterial systems studied appears to be closely linked on a chromosome
to the operon that it controls and since its influence appears to be
exerted only over short distances, the hypothetical operators introduced
into the hybrid by the normal chromosome complement would not
affect the functioning of comparable operons of the tumor chromosomes. This could lead to the continued synthesis in the hybrid cell
of specific proteins. Yet the deletion hypotheses are not concerned
with the synthesis of new proteins but rather with the persistent
deletion of certain normally synthesized proteins.

The results of hybridization are also incompatible with any hypothesis based on recessive mutations. It would, nevertheless, be most
interesting to hybridize tumor cells in which deletions are strongly
suspected of being etiologically involved, such as, for example, malig-

nant cell types found in chronic myelocytic leukemia, with their normal counterparts to learn whether in those instances the tumor or normal properties were dominant.

Deletions Other than Those Involved Etiologically. The results of the hybridization studies do not, of course, mean that deletions other than those etiologically involved in establishing the cancerous state may not occur. Such deletions would be placed in the "non-essential" category by Potter. An interesting example of this would appear to be found in certain lymphosarcomas and leukemias, the cells of which have presumably lost the ability to synthesize asparagine but which require that substance for growth.

In 1953 Kidd (280) observed that certain transplanted murine leukemias were suppressed by treatment with guinea pig serum. The active component in the guinea pig serum was found by Broome (94) to be the enzyme L-asparaginase. By treating mice with certain leukemias (73), dogs with lymphosarcomas (387), and humans with certain leukemias (386) with L-asparaginase, dramatic remissions have been obtained.

The cells of tumors that respond to L-asparaginase require L-asparagine for growth while normal cells and cells of insensitive tumors are independent of an external source of this amino acid. The effectiveness of L-asparaginase as a chemotherapeutic agent depends then upon a specific metabolic defect in certain malignant cells.

Addition of New Genetic Information

In contrast to the dearth of definitive information concerning the deletion of genetic information in the establishment of the neoplastic state, the evidence for the addition of new information resulting from infection by the oncogenic viruses appears unequivocal. The oncogenic viruses, like the generality of viruses, may be either RNA-containing, as in the case of the Rous sarcoma virus or the wound tumor virus of plants, or DNA-containing, of which the polyoma virus, the simian vacuolating virus (SV40), and certain of the adenoviruses may be considered as prototypes.

The oncogenic viruses as a group offer an unusually promising model for studying *in vitro* cellular changes leading to the neoplastic transformation. Few other kinds of carcinogenic agents provoke so direct and immediate a response and for no other type of carcinogen are the possibilities of the interaction of the provoking agent with cellular mechanisms so extensive.

A number of *in vitro* systems have been developed for a study of the oncogenic viruses. Extensive information is available on the action of the polyoma virus and the SV40 virus in monolayer cultures of mouse and hamster cells as well as on the action of the Rous sarcoma virus in monolayers of chick cells. These agents give rise to profound cellular changes which have been extensively reviewed.

The RNA-containing Viruses.

The Rous sarcoma virus. Although the Rous agent in chickens was among the first of the tumor-inducing viruses to be discovered, little progress was made for many years in gaining an understanding of the viral-host cell interaction. This was largely due to the unavailability of a simple quantitative assay method. Following the initial studies by Halberstaedter et al. (225) and those of Manaker and Groupé (336), Rubin and Temin developed a quantitative assay and used the technique for the determination of virus as well as for the registration of Rous-virus-infected cells (431, 433, 512).

With the development of such an assay system, progress has been made over the past decade in an understanding of the viral-host cell interaction in the Rous sarcoma system.

The Rous sarcoma virus is a medium-sized leukovirus that contains a single-stranded RNA molecule which is combined with a large number of protein subunits, all of which are contained in a special outer membrane composed of both protein and lipid. The viral RNA has a molecular weight of about 10 million composed of 30,000 nucleotides. About 10,000 amino acids are thus coded for by the Rous virus genome, a number sufficient for the production of at least 25 new proteins. The very recent studies of Duesberg (158) suggest that the Rous virus RNA may be significantly smaller than the earlier studies indicated.

It has been found in the case of the Rous sarcoma virus, in contrast to certain of the DNA-containing oncogenic viruses to be described later in this chapter, that chick cells transformed *in vitro* synthesize virus continuously. Studies with the use of certain strains of the Rous sarcoma virus have been complicated, however, because of the consistent association of certain other leukosis viruses. An analysis of the interaction of these viruses led originally to the erroneous assumption that some strains of the Rous sarcoma virus are dependent upon associated leukosis viruses for their reproduction and those strains of the Rous virus were therefore considered to be defective. More recent studies have shown that transformed chick cells do produce infectious virus whose host range is, however, severely restricted. This is not the case with mammalian cells transformed by the Rous virus. In that instance infectious virus can only be recovered when the transformed cells are cultivated in the presence of normal chick cells.

The description of the Rous sarcoma virus as a defective virus was based on the belief that it was unable to form its own coat and that it relied on a helper virus for that function. Dougherty and Di Stefano (156) examined the ultrastructure of "non-virus-producing" transformed cells and found virus particles that were indistinguishable from typical Rous sarcoma virus particles to be present at the surface of such cells. This contradiction was soon resolved when Vogt (532) found that Rous sarcoma virus produced from "nonproducing" transformed cells had a limited host range. While this virus was essentially noninfectious in cells derived from C/O type chick embryos, the type most commonly used, it was found to be infectious in cells derived from C/A type. The most susceptible cell type was shown to be the Japanese quail embryo cell. It now seems clear, therefore, that the Rous sarcoma virus does produce a significant number of virus particles which are infectious for certain host cells without the aid of a helper virus and it is therefore not defective in any viral function. The role of the helper virus is to extend the limited host range of the Rous virus by contributing its coat material to the Rous particle.

The central problem in tumorigenesis with the Rous agent is the exact form of the association that develops between the virus and the target cell.

Despite the fact that transformations by RNA viruses would appear to imply mechanisms below the gene or chromosome levels, there were repeated early suggestions that viral and host cell genomes might be linked in a manner comparable to that found in the lysogenic state in the bacteria (159, 160, 406, 430, 431). More recently, Temin (506, 508) has presented evidence that appears to indicate that a curious relationship of the viral genome with a host cell chromosome may, in fact, occur. It was found by Temin that, unlike most other RNA viruses, the initial synthesis of the Rous sarcoma virus in an infected cell apparently required the action as well as the synthesis of host cell DNA. These findings, which have been confirmed by others (23, 24, 528), may be interpreted to mean that after entry into a cell the RNA of the Rous sarcoma virus is used as a template to form a complementary DNA strand. In accord with this hypothesis, the DNA strand, presumably after formation of a subsequent complementary DNA strand, is inserted into a host cell chromosome where it replicates with the DNA of the host. In support of this interpretation Temin (507) has shown that DNA isolated from Rous-sarcoma-virus-infected cells contains a small region in which one of its chains is complementary in sequence to Rous sarcoma virus RNA. No such homology was found when hybridization studies were similarly made with uninfected cells.

These findings suggest an RNA to DNA transfer of information and that the replicating form of the virus may, in fact, be an RNA-DNA hybrid. Further evidence consistent with the idea that a DNA-RNA hybrid molecule may play a role in the replication of Rous sarcoma virus has been provided by the observation that Rous-infected cells contain complexes in which high molecular weight viral RNA is largely RNase-resistant. This RNase-resistant state is abolished by the action of DNase (408). This is, nevertheless, clearly a radical proposal and more evidence would appear to be needed before it gains general acceptance. At any rate, such a DNA provirus, which is postulated to be integrated into the DNA of the host cell nucleus and which serves as a template for viral RNA synthesis, cannot be integrated in any very stable fashion since, as Macpherson (330) has shown, significant numbers of progeny of cloned transformed hamster cells recover from the tumorous state apparently as a result of the loss of the viral and, by implication, the proviral genome from the cell.

Studies with the use of the Schmidt-Ruppin strain of the Rous sarcoma virus indicate that only a portion of its genome is needed for transformation since oncogenesis and infectivity can be dissociated by irradiation (206). Superinfection with avian leukosis virus of "non-producer" cells transformed by the irradiated virus does not lead to the release of infective virus.

Although, as indicated earlier, enough new genetic information is introduced into a Rous-virus-infected cell to code for at least ten proteins, little is as yet known concerning the nature of the viral associated functions. It has, however, been shown (6, 172, 509) that the conversion of cell morphology induced by the Rous sarcoma virus is associated with an increased rate of acid mucopolysaccharide production. This increased synthesis is associated with a two- to sixfold increase in the level of an enzyme involved in acid muco-polysaccharide production. Huebner et al. (252) have found, moreover, that tumors of hamsters and guinea pigs induced by the Schmidt-Ruppin strain of the Rous sarcoma virus contain new specific antigens but do not produce the infectious virus. It is interesting to speculate that the induction of new proteins could render viruses tumorigenic if the protein in question served to trigger continued cell proliferation. Thus, a virus-induced protein of an appropriate type might provide the mitotic stimulus for enduring malignant growth.

Black's wound tumor disease virus. Black's wound tumor disease of plants is also caused by an RNA-containing virus that is well characterized. The virus replicates in its insect vector as well as in susceptible plant species. The host range of the virus is large and some 43 plant species in 20 different families have been found to support replication of the virus. In some host species such as sweet clover (*Melilotus alba* Desr.) and sorrel (*Rumex acetosa* L.) the response to infection involves the formation of tumors. Such tumors show a capacity for unlimited growth both *in vivo* and *in vitro*. Although this disease is caused by a virus and the virus is systemic in the host, tumor inception and development are limited to areas of irritation such as those resulting from a wound, increased hormone levels, etc. In addition to the virus and an area of irritation, the genetic constitution of the host plays an important role in the expression of the disease.

The wound tumor virus has been isolated, pictured with the aid of an electron microscope, and found to be a polyhedron having a diameter of about 60 mμ. The virus has an internal core of double-stranded RNA that has a molecular weight of about 15 million. There appear to be 92 capsomeres present in the protein coat of the virus. The wound tumor virus thus resembles the reoviruses in morphology. Black (59) has reported that there is about 50 times as much nucleic acid in a single strand of the double-stranded RNA of the virus as is required for the synthesis of the protein coat. Since the single strand of RNA can code for approximately 7,500 amino acids, it is evident that the RNA contains genetic information sufficient to code for more than ten viral functions. Except for information required for the synthesis of viral coat protein, none of these functions has as yet been characterized.

It is, nevertheless, clear that in this instance, as in the case of crown gall neoplasms, the tumor cells are significantly less fastidious in their nutritional requirements than are their normal counterparts. The tumor cells have acquired as a result of viral infection the capacity to synthesize all of the essential metabolites that they require for their continued cell growth and division from mineral salts, sucrose, and three vitamins. It appears unlikely that the genetic information introduced into a cell by the virus codes specifically for the two hormones, the auxins and the cytokinins, as well as for the other essential metabolites that are required for continued cell growth and division. It would appear more reasonable to assume that, in this instance, the virus brings about a derepression of the host cell genome and that this, in turn, results in the synthesis by the tumor cell of the essential metabolites. Just how such a derepression could be accomplished in this system is not yet clear.

The DNA-containing Viruses. In considering the DNA-containing viruses, the small papovaviruses, of which the polyoma and SV40 viruses are prototypes, may be used as models since they have been most thoroughly studied. The DNA carried by these viruses is of a circular, double-stranded type which is enclosed in a protein coat. Infection of cells by these viruses is of two types, the productive type in which the virus multiplies essentially unchecked and eventually lyses and kills the cells, and the abortive type in which there is little or no productive infection but there is instead a transformation leading to the tumorous state. Transformations occur with a rather low frequency in such systems.

Virus-cell interactions. When suitable cells are infected with the polyoma virus, a large number of viral particles accumulate around the nucleus of the cell. Most of these particles remain unchanged but in some instances the protein coat is removed and the naked

DNA enters the nucleus. There are essentially two lines of evidence which indicate that the transformation process is caused by the viral DNA and the genes that it carries.

The first of these is concerned with the fact that transformation can be achieved with the use of purified viral DNA (153). The protein of the viral coat does not, on the other hand, transform cells. That the transforming ability of the viral DNA does not reside in some contaminant carried by the isolated DNA was demonstrated by workers at the University of Glasgow. It has been found that viral DNA may in some instances be contaminated with cellular DNA. The DNA of the papovaviruses is found in the form of ring-shaped supercoils. If one of the strands suffers a single break, the supercoil disappears and the molecule becomes a stretched ring in solution. These two molecular types can be separated into two distinct bands with density-gradient centrifugation techniques. Examination of the biological properties of such preparations showed that the transforming ability as well as productive infection is strictly limited to the two bands of the viral DNA. These findings rule out the possibility that transforming ability is due to contaminating fragments of cellular DNA since the contaminating molecules have a very different distribution in the gradient.

A second type of evidence that demonstrates that the function of the viral genome is required for transformation is found in the experiments of Fried (189) who studied a temperature-sensitive mutant of the polyoma virus Ts-a. This mutant behaves like the normal virus at 31°C. At 39°C, on the other hand, the virus is unable to cause either a transformation or a productive infection, thus demonstrating that a mutation in the viral DNA can abolish the ability of the virus to transform cells.

The question that arises next, therefore, is whether continued presence of the viral genome is required for the continued abnormal proliferation of the transformed cell or whether the viral genome, once it exerts its effects, is no longer required for the continued abnormal growth of the tumor cells. The second possibility requires careful consideration because one of the early events following cellular transformation by the polyoma virus is the development of chromosome breaks leading to abnormal karyotypes. Yet, as indicated above, chromosome breaks do not appear to be the mechanism underlying tumor-igenesis in this system.

It is, nevertheless, well known that cells transformed by polyoma or SV40 viruses carry all or part of the viral genome for many cell generations without ever producing coat protein or the complete virus. The continued presence of the viral genome in transformed cells can be demonstrated in several ways. This is evidenced first by the fact that a virus coded antigen which is found in nuclei of lytically infected cells is also found in nuclei of transformed cells. This antigen, called the T (tumor) antigen, has been demonstrated by immuno-fluorescence and complement fixation techniques. It has been shown (47, 190), moreover, with nucleic acid hybridization studies that transformed cells contain virus-specific ribonucleic acid, thus indicating, with the use of this very sensitive and specific method, the presence in the cells of functional viral DNA. This idea has received further support by the finding that cells of certain clonal cell lines transformed by either the polyoma virus or SV40 are very different in appearance. Results such as these can perhaps best be explained by assuming that the differences that accompany transformation by the two viruses are the result of two different viral genomes functioning in different cells of the same cell type.

Finally, it has been demonstrated by means of cell fusion studies (541, 296) that complete virus may, in fact, be produced by certain cells transformed by the SV40 virus. These studies suggest that the presence of the viral genome is necessary for the maintenance of the neoplastic state. However, as will be indicated later, the presence of the viral genome may not in itself be sufficient to account for the existence of the transformed state (399). As Dulbecco points out (161), a conclusive clarification of the role of persisting viral genes could be obtained by using temperature-dependent viral mutants in which the mutation of a gene, whose function is necessary for maintaining the cells in the transformed state, would cause transformation at low temperature but that such transformed cells would revert to normal when the ambient temperature was raised. Although such mutants are being actively searched for, none have been described at the time of this writing.

This problem has been approached experimentally in another way by making use of a phenomenon known as anchorage-dependence in

BHK21 cells infected with polyoma virus (489). When such cells were planted in an agar-containing medium with transforming virus, the usual small percentage ranging from 1% to 5% of the cells was transformed. When, on the other hand, such cells were similarly planted into a viscous solution of "Methacel," one-third to one-half of the cells appeared to have been transformed since they formed colonies in the "Methacel"-containing medium. When, however, such colony-forming cells were removed and cultured further, the majority reverted to normal. It was concluded by Stoker that the transformation may either be temporary, in which case the cells become normal again when the virus is lost, or be permanent if the viral DNA is integrated into the genome of the host cell. It was suggested further that, although the physiology of the transformed cell does not depend on integration, transformation can be perpetuated only if the viral DNA is integrated. There is evidence that the viral genome or a part of it persists and continues to be transcribed in cells derived from tumors induced by human adenovirus 12 (190). There is now also evidence for linkage between the genome of adenovirus 12, or a part of it, and the cellular DNA (154).

It has been found, moreover, by means of a modified DNA-RNA hybridization technique that nuclei of cells transformed by either polyoma or SV40 contain viral DNA (552). In a continuation of these studies (441), using the SV40-virus-transformed 3T3 cells, it was found that the transformed cells contain twenty SV40 DNA equivalents per cell. It was also found that the viral DNA molecules are integrated with cell DNA by alkali-stable covalent linkages. It was not determined in those studies whether the viral DNA is linked to the cellular DNA in one large piece at a single locus or whether it is connected at multiple sites following many individual insertions.

Viral functions. The DNA of the small papovaviruses has a molecular weight of about 3 million and each DNA strand contains about 5,000 bases. Since 3 bases are required to specify 1 amino acid in a polypeptide chain, it follows that 5,000 bases can specify some 1,700 amino acids. It can be calculated, moreover, from the molecular weight of the protein coat and the number of subunits found therein that between one-third and one-fourth of the genetic information of the virus is required to specify the coat protein. The remaining genetic information, which can specify about 1,200 amino acids, is adequate to code for between 4 and 8 new proteins depending on their size. This is, therefore, the maximum number of viral genetic functions that can be involved in the transformation process. Genetic information specifying coat protein is irrelevant, as we have seen, because no coat protein is synthesized in transformed cells.

By comparing normal cells, productively infected cells, and transformed cells it has now been possible to specify seven functions that have been identified with virus activity. These studies have not as yet been carried far enough to be certain that each new cellular function represents the activity of a separate viral gene or whether all of the gene functions have, in fact, been identified. Nevertheless, of the seven viral functions that have thus far been specified, two or three are particularly suspect as being critically involved in the transformation process. The first of these is a virus-specific antigen that is present on the surface of transformed cells. This antigen, which is known as the transplantation antigen, was detected independently by Sjögren et al. (454) and Habel (221). These workers found that if an animal is, for example, immunized with the polyoma virus, it will reject cells transformed by that virus but not cells transformed by the SV40 virus. The reverse is also true. Thus the antigen is virus-specific. It has been suggested that since this new antigen is a surface antigen it may be responsible for the loss of contact relations shown by the transformed cells.

A second interesting and perhaps highly significant cellular function identified with viral activity is the activation of the synthesis of cellular DNA and of the enzymes required for that synthesis. It is clear that if the viral gene responsible for this activating function persists and operates in transformed cells, it could very well make such cells insensitive to the mechanisms that normally regulate growth. However, direct evidence for such a regulatory mechanism involving a derepression of the genome has not yet been obtained.

A third viral function which may well be associated with gene activation is the synthesis of a virus-specific antigen known as the T or tumor antigen. This antigen differs in immunological specificity from both the surface or transplantation antigen and the viral coat protein antigen. The T antigen is present in the nucleus of both transformed and productively infected cells. That the T antigen may represent a protein with a regulatory function is suggested by the observation that it appears before either the induction of cellular DNA synthesis or the replication of the viral DNA. However, in view of the studies of Pollack et al. (399), it appears likely that although the T antigen may be necessary it is not in itself sufficient to maintain the neoplastic state.

A fourth viral function is concerned with the gene bearing the Ts-a mutation which, it will be recalled, leads to a defective virus that can bring about a transformation at 31°C but not at 39°C. Cells transformed at the lower temperature remain transformed when placed at the higher temperature. Thus, the function of the Ts-a gene may not be directly involved or may be only transiently required in the transformation process.

The last three viral functions that have been described do not appear to be directly related to the transformation process. The first of these is concerned with the synthesis by productively infected cells of a thymidine kinase that is different from the enzyme normally produced by the cell. This viral induced thymidine kinase has not, as yet, been found in transformed cells and its induction may, therefore, be associated entirely with productive infection. A second new function not directly related to transformation and observed so far only with the SV40 virus is that after cells have been productively infected with that virus they become susceptible to an adenovirus, the replication of which they do not normally support. Finally, a third new viral function in productively infected cells is the specification of viral coat protein. Since this coat protein is not synthesized in transformed cells, the genes specifying its synthesis must either be absent or be silent. That the latter is probably true is suggested, at least in the case of the SV40 virus, by the finding that complete virus may be produced by the transformed cells as a result of cell fusion.

Unless some few viral functions remain uncharacterized, it would appear that the central mechanism of cancer induction in the two instances described above resides in possibly two such functions. The problem is thus narrowly restricted and there is every reason to believe that the questionable points still remaining will be resolved in the near future. There are, nevertheless, three possibilities that must clearly be kept in mind when attempting to interpret the results described above. The first of these, as already indicated, is that the viral nucleic acids exert their oncogenic effects by virtue of their function as templates for the synthesis of new and specific products which are, in turn, directly responsible for the establishment and maintenance of the tumorous state. Alternatively, these new and specific products derived from the activities of the viral genome may be exerting their biological effects indirectly by bringing about a persistent activation of that segment of the host cell genome that is concerned with cell growth and division. In this instance the newly synthesized products responsible for the autonomous proliferation of the tumor cells would be coded for not by viral genes but by the genome of the host cell. Finally, the viral nucleic acids may derepress host cell functions by means other than those involving transcription and translation of the viral genome.

The thoughts presented above concerning the DNA-containing oncogenic viruses are in part those expressed by Dulbecco (161).

CHAPTER V

Other Types of
Heritable Cellular Change

Extrachromosomal Heredity in Lower Forms

The question that arises next is, Can a heritable change in the phenotype occur without a corresponding change in the integrity of the genotype? If the answer to that question is No, then carcinogenesis must clearly involve somatic mutation at the nuclear gene level. If, on the other hand, an affirmative answer can be provided experimentally, then quite different mechanisms can be envisioned for the origin of a cancer cell.

The answer to the question posed above is, of course, Yes. Heritable changes in the phenotype can occur without corresponding changes in the genotype. Numerous examples of extrachromosomal inheritance are documented in two recently published books (268, 557). Such types of non-Mendelian heredity have been described, among others, in the fungi (476), in the algae (438), and in the Protozoa. The diversity of the cellular mechanisms that may underlie such heritable changes is well illustrated in the case of the *Paramecium*. Here we find the "killer" phenomenon which is dependent upon the presence of a DNA-containing parasite (465), cortical inheritance which is independent of the genome and is determined by pre-existing structure (466), the Dauermodifications of Jollos (270) which are concerned with the non-Mendelian inheritance of an acquired tolerance to certain toxic substances, as well as the familiar alternative serotypes that are found in that organism (42). It may be suggested, however, that certain of the hereditary phenomena that have been designated as non-Mendelian may, in fact, be epigenetic in that the primary genetic information accounting for such types of heredity may ultimately be found to reside in the chromosomes.

Somatic Cell Heredity in Higher Forms

Topophysis or Phase Change in Higher Plants

The several examples cited above have dealt entirely with lower forms. Are there, then, examples of discontinuous but potentially reversible heritable changes found in higher organisms? Examples of this type of somatic cell heredity are well illustrated in a phenomenon that has been termed topophysis or phase change and that is characteristic of many higher plant species and that, according to Brink (92), has its counterpart in the animal field as well.

During the course of development, the apical meristems of many different higher plants may undergo an abrupt or, less frequently, a gradual switch in potential from that characteristic of the juvenile stage of a plant species to that distinctive of the adult type of growth. Such changes are often marked by pronounced changes in phenotypic expression. This is illustrated in Figure 7 in which the juvenile and adult forms of *Acacia* are shown. The English ivy *Hedera helix* represents another classical example of phase change in woody plant species. The juvenile form of this species is a trailing or climbing vine with dorsiventral symmetry, palmately lobed leaves, and 2/2 phyllotaxy. This form is sterile. The adult form, on the other hand, is a semi-erect or erect shrub with entire ovate leaves and 2/5 phyllotaxy. The adult form is fertile.

When seeds derived from the adult form are planted they invariably give rise to juvenile plants. It is thus clear that a phase reversal from the adult to the juvenile stage always follows sexual reproduction. Yet cuttings derived from either juvenile or adult shoots which may be found on the same plant retain their respective characteristics often for many years.

Although spontaneous phase reversal in adult ivy appears to be a very rare event in nature, rejuvenation has been accomplished experimentally in a number of different ways. For example, Frank and Renner (188) reported that if buds found on adult branches were

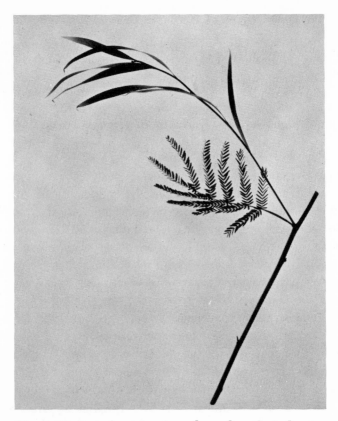

Fig. 7. Portion of an *Acacia melanoxylon* plant showing juvenile and adult forms of growth. The phyllode pattern of growth is shown developing from the axil of a compound leaf. This material illustrates very well the fact that striking changes may occur in the phenotype without a corresponding change in the genotype. (Courtesy of Dr. William J. Robbins.)

treated with X-irradiation, the resulting shoots scored 7 months later bore leaves characteristic of the juvenile stage. These investigators also observed that new branches that developed from adult ivy cuttings treated at −10°C for 3 to 4 hours were typically juvenile in character. Robbins (415) found that repeated spraying of adult *Hedera canariensis variegata* plants with gibberellic acid over a 19-week period resulted in the development of juvenile branches from some of the plants. These findings were later confirmed by Robbins with the use of *Hedera helix* (416). In this latter paper Robbins also reported that new shoots formed on severely and repeatedly pruned adult plants of English ivy were fully juvenile in some instances and intermediate in others. This investigator emphasized the fact that the observed juvenile shoots could not have come from buds that were in the juvenile state prior to pruning because the new shoots showed progression from the adult condition at the base to the juvenile state toward the tip. Thus although the transition from adult to juvenile and juvenile to adult is commonly abrupt, it may in some instances be gradual.

Doorenbos (155) observed intermediate forms during the transition from juvenile to adult, while Kranz (297) found that cuttings taken from a transitional zone retained their intermediate characteristics over long periods of time. The finding of stable intermediates is very reminiscent of the type of graded series of stable changes found in the crown gall tumor system in plants as well as in tumor progressions found in animals. It is interesting to note that when juvenile and adult ivy tissues are isolated sterilely and cultured in the same environment, pronounced differences in their growth patterns are observed. Tissue from the adult form grows very slowly and in a compact manner, while that isolated from the juvenile form grows rapidly and is friable, and commonly forms roots (495). These characteristic growth patterns appear to be retained indefinitely in culture, thus apparently reflecting profound inherent differences in the two kinds of tissue.

Brink (92) has deduced certain generalizations concerning the process of phase change, some of which are listed below:

1. Phase change occurs in somatic cells, and is a conspicuous feature of development in many species of higher plants.
2. Alternative phases, in some cases, differ sharply in phenotype, but change from one phase to the other may involve transitional phenotypes.
3. Phase change is reversible under certain physiological conditions.
4. Change from one phase to the other is a directed response to stimuli originating outside the affected apical meristem.
5. Once established, a given growth phase tends to be constant under continuous vegetative propagation, even in the absence of the environmental factor which incited it.

6. The frequency of phase change, however, is far higher than that characteristic of germinally transmissible mutations.

7. Phase change is associated with meristematic growth, not with aging of quiescent meristems.

8. The reversal of phase, which invariably occurs during sexual reproduction, is not directly attributable to either meiosis or fertilization, as genetic processes.

Brink has pointed out that counterparts of phase change, expressed in a wide variety of ways, are common among both plants and animals. This phenomenon illustrates a general aspect of somatic cell heredity in which, despite striking differences in phenotypic expression, the genotype remains constant. Phase change appears, then, to be merely one manifestation of the larger problem of cellular differentiation and development which will be considered in detail next.

Cellular Differentiation

One of the most commonly found types of heritable change that does not appear, in most instances at least, to involve a change in the integrity of the genetic information present in a cell is that concerned with cellular differentiation in the normal course of development. Attempts to elucidate the mechanism(s) underlying cellular differentiation have had a long and often tortured history. It was assumed for many years that all of the genes in every cell were active all of the time. Hence, it seemed meaningless to consider direct gene action as relevant to problems of cellular differentiation since that phenomenon is characterized by the fact that it results in the production of different kinds of cells. Attention was therefore directed toward the cytoplasm since, although the genes were believed to remain the same, the cytoplasm varied. Yet it was known that almost every step in the development of such a well-studied organism as the common fruit fly *Drosophila* was modifiable by mutation at the nuclear gene level. It was thus recognized that the genes as well as the cytoplasm must somehow be involved.

This dilemma was finally resolved about twenty-five years ago when evidence began to accumulate from a number of directions for the presence of active and inactive gene states in the chromosomes. Perhaps no study was more influential in establishing this concept than that of Monod and his collaborators on the genetic control of the enzyme β-galactosidase in the bacterium *Escherichia coli*. This classic series of studies, which will be considered in Chapter VII, has in the past and continues to provide model systems for the control of gene action not only in the bacteria but in higher organisms as well.

It is now believed that most of the genetic information found in a cell is repressed and hence nonfunctional and that different genes are responsive to different specific signals that derepress them and regulate their activities. Thus, differences among cells with identical sets of genes could be due to the activity of different genes in different types of cells. With a model such as this it is easy to understand why, for example, erythrocytes synthesize hemoglobin while lymphocytes do not, why kidney cells produce L amino acid oxidase while liver cells do not but instead synthesize, as a product of their differentiation, serum albumin. Since it now appears that many genes remain nonfunctional unless specifically derepressed, the synthesis of different proteins in different cell types would appear to depend upon the presence of specific substances that derepress them. Variable gene activity is, then, the guiding principle upon which much of the current research in the field of cellular differentiation is based. Unfortunately, theory in this area is far ahead of knowledge and the mechanisms that control differential gene activity are just beginning to be explored (467).

Evidence for Selective Gene Activation. What, then, is the evidence upon which this powerful and provocative concept is based for organisms higher in the evolutionary scale than are the bacteria? That different somatic cells within an organism carry equivalent genetic endowments is suggested by the equivalence of chromosome numbers in diploid cells present in various specialized tissues of such organisms. This is, moreover, established at a chemical level by the findings of Mirsky and Ris (361) as well as of the Vendrelys (527) who reported that diploid nuclei of different somatic cells of an organism commonly contain equal or nearly equal amounts of DNA per nucleus while haploid gametes contain half as much. The elegant experiments of McCarthy and Hoyer (348) have demonstrated, furthermore, the identity of DNA and the diversity of rapidly labeled RNA in cells of different tissues of the mouse. Since DNA is firmly established as the carrier of genetic information, these findings support the concept of the maintenance of a full genome in differentiated cells of many kinds. It is perfectly clear, moreover, that the diploid progenitor of the haploid gamete must contain all of the genes present in the antecedent zygote.

There are, furthermore, certain types of cells whose developmental potentialities would be difficult to explain without the assumption of the presence in those cells of a full complement of genes. For example, differentiated somatic cells of certain higher plant species are capable, when placed in a favorable environment, of developing into a complete organism (483, 525). Animals of some of the lower phyla are not much less versatile than are plants since an entire organism can in many instances regenerate from a small fragment of tissue.

Developmental potentialities of transplant nuclei. Equally striking are the results reported by Gurdon and Uehlinger (220) who demonstrated that nuclei taken from differentiated intestinal epithelial cells of feeding tadpoles of the African clawed toad *Xenopus laevis* when implanted into eggs of the same species were capable in some instances of supporting the development of completely normal fertile adult animals. Although in *Xenopus,* as in *Rana pipiens* to be described below, the ability of transfer nuclei to promote normal differentiation declines with age, a number of normal embryos have been obtained with nuclei from remarkably advanced stages of development. These positive results include the development of typical larvae by implantation into eggs of nuclei from endoderm and mesoderm, of neural fold, tailbud, and even the muscular response stage. All of these findings indicate that certain nuclei at least may remain totipotent well beyond the time when cellular differentiation is expressed morphologically.

The capacity of certain vertebrates to restore lost parts such as limbs and tails through regeneration also supports arguments in favor of the presence of most if not the full informational content in nuclei of the regenerating cells. This matter will be discussed in greater detail below.

Despite evidence of the type cited above, the maintenance of the full genome in differentiated cells of higher animals still lacks final proof. A most obvious exception to this concept as a generalization is the mature red blood cell of man which lacks a nucleus and hence has lost all of its nuclear DNA. There are other exceptions. In the case of *Ascaris* (68) and *Sciara* (355), differentiation is regularly associated with the loss of parts of chromosomes and the more recent studies (31, 328) on sex-linked characters in mammals have indicated that an irreversible change occurs in the X chromosome which becomes cytologically compact and genetically inactive at the time of gastrulation. These examples, however, represent special cases and do not appear to affect significantly the validity of the concept of nuclear equivalence during development.

The studies of Briggs and King and their associates do, however, raise some questions regarding this matter. These workers transplanted nuclei from cells of the frog *Rana pipiens* in various periods of development into enucleated frog eggs and found that nuclei from fairly early stages commonly supported normal development while those of later stages did not. Thus, King and Briggs (286, 287) reported that more than one-half of the eggs that had received nuclei from the blastula or early gastrula stage cleaved normally and more than 85% of those developed into normal larvae. Quite different results were obtained when donor nuclei were taken from chordamesoderm or from presumptive medullary plate of the late gastrula. In both instances development of the recipient eggs is much more restricted. Cleavage occurs in only a minority of implanted eggs and further development of such embryos is abnormal. About half stop developing as blastulae or gastrulae, while the majority of others arrest at the neurula or postneurula stages (286, 287).

That the nuclei become specialized as development proceeds and lose progressively their capacity to promote the full range of developmental processes is suggested by further studies of Briggs and King (88, 90). It was found in those investigations that when nuclei taken from the midgut at the end of gastrulation were implanted into competent eggs, the majority gave rise to defective embryos. The observed deficiencies appeared, moreover, to reflect the developmental fate of the donor nuclei. Although most of these embryos were deficient in ectodermal derivatives, structures formed from endoderm appeared normal and both notochord and somites were found to be present. It should be noted that a nuclear clone derived from nuclei of a first transplant blastula develops more uniformly than the original transplant generation. Although marked differences in developmental patterns are observed between different clones, the patterns within any one clone are remarkably stable (288).

Central to all of these findings is the nature of the restrictions that appear progressively as nuclear differentiation of the embryo proceeds. These changes appear to be stable and perhaps even irreversible. One possibility, suggested by the studies of Briggs, King, and DiBerardino (91, 151), is that chromosomal aberrations may be involved. Briggs and King (89) suggested earlier that the loss of some closely associated perinuclear organelle in the cytoplasm cannot be ruled out as having a causal relationship. Alternatively, and perhaps more probably, nuclear differentiation merely involves stable shifts in the functional states of the genes present in the nuclei. Thus, in the instance cited above in which the embryos were deficient in ectodermal but not in endodermal derivatives the nuclei may have been potentially totipotent but as a result of nuclear differentiation the genes concerned with ectodermal development, although present, were repressed. Unfortunately, these studies were complicated by the fact that chromosomal aberrations were present and the extent of these deficiencies was found to be directly related to the degree of development obtained.

Developmental potentialities of Lucké tumor nuclei. In a continuation of the nuclear transplant work, nuclei from the Lucké renal cell carcinoma of the frog were placed into enucleated frog eggs in order to determine the developmental potentialities of the tumor nuclei. The Lucké adenocarcinoma is a malignant tumor that is almost certainly of viral origin, as indicated earlier. Cytologically, tumors of the Lucké type have a comparatively normal chromosome complement and analysis of tumors maintained for over two years by means of serial transfer showed few departures from the normal diploid karyotype (152). When nuclei of the adenocarcinoma were transplanted into enucleated eggs, remarkable results were obtained. Not only did the nuclei participate in normal cleavage, but some of the eggs also formed complete gastrulae and a few exceptional specimens even developed into abnormal postneurula and swimming-stage larvae.

Histological analysis by McKinnell (352) of tumor nuclear transplants which attained late embryonic stages showed that although the heart and optic cup developed abnormally, all other organs examined showed good histogenesis. More recently, DiBerardino and King (151) found that all organs developed abnormally. They attributed this variance to differences in the karyotypes of the euploid embryos obtained by McKinnell and by themselves. These workers also compared the developmental potentialities of tumor nuclei and normal kidney cell nuclei and found that developmentally they behaved similarly and possessed similar types of nuclear abnormalities.

These findings are of considerable significance as far as the biology of the cancer problem is concerned. Most striking was the absence of any evidence of malignancy in embryos containing tumor nuclei despite the common occurrence of aneuploid karyotypes. It is thus apparent that the nuclei of these tumor cells are not irreversibly altered. When tumor nuclei are placed in the proper cytoplasmic environment the cells are no longer capable of progressive uncontrolled cell division but, rather, such nuclei respond beautifully to the mechanisms that normally control those processes. These studies demonstrate, moreover, that the genomic information present in the tumor nuclei has been conserved sufficiently to enable the embryos to form all of the cell types of the differentiated organ systems found in control larvae of the same age. Since this tumor is almost certainly caused by a virus, another important implication of these studies would appear to be that this oncogenic virus, at least, does not irreversibly alter the genetic information of the cell that leads to the development of the neoplastic state.

Biochemical evidence for selective gene activation. It is now firmly established that the synthesis of the several classes of RNA's in the nucleus is DNA-dependent. It is, nevertheless, important to stress that only a relatively small part of the total chromosomal DNA is actually functioning as a template for RNA synthesis at any one time. This fact was demonstrated experimentally by progressively removing DNA from nuclei with the use of increasing concentrations of the enzyme DNase. The effects of DNA depletion on nuclear function were then tested (16, 18). The results of those studies showed that between 70% and 80% and possibly more of the DNA could be removed from nuclei with no significant effect on the amount of RNA synthesized. It was found, however, that if the remainder of the DNA was removed enzymatically, RNA synthesis came to an abrupt halt. If, on the other hand, only a portion of the remaining DNA was removed the rate of RNA synthesis decreased proportionately. Thus, a linear correspondence between the amount of DNA remaining in the nucleus and its ability to synthesize RNA was found (16).

It was, therefore, concluded from those studies that almost all of the DNA removed must have been nonfunctional as far as RNA synthesis is concerned and that only a small part of the total was available as a template for the RNA polymerase reaction.

Electron microscopic evidence with the use of lymphocyte nuclei revealed that the chromatin is distributed in dense clumps of compacted fibrils and in diffuse regions of extended filaments having 100 to 150 Å diameters (312, 314). Electron density studies of these nuclear areas following uranyl acetate staining showed a close correspondence to their DNA content, as visualized by Feulgen staining of matching thick sections (312). From such comparisons it was concluded that most of the DNA of the nucleus is found in the electron-dense areas, while the diffuse chromatin contains only a small fraction of the total DNA. These studies were pursued further by studying the biosynthetic activity directly with the use of high-resolution auto-radiography (312, 114). The results of those studies demonstrated that most of the uridine ^{3}H label was found over or very close to the regions of diffuse chromatin, while but few grains were seen over the large masses of condensed chromatin. It clearly follows, therefore, that most of the DNA in the nucleus is inactive in promoting RNA synthesis. These conclusions are in accord with those of others (211) who have reported that RNA synthesis occurs preferentially in the diffuse chromatin of kidney cell nuclei.

Visible evidence for selective gene activation. Perhaps the most convincing visible evidence that genes of higher organisms are differentially activated and repressed in cells of different tissues has come from studies of two types of unusually large chromosomes, the lamp-brush chromosomes of amphibian oocytes and the giant polytene chromosomes of certain Diptera such as *Drosophila, Chironomus, Sciara,* and *Rhynchosciara.* This fascinating subject has been extensively reviewed by Beermann (45), Clever (122), Davidson and Mirsky (142), Gall (191), and Pavan (390).

Lampbrush chromosomes are found in growing oocytes and spermatocytes of many organisms during the so-called diplotene stage of meiotic prophase. Their occurrence is correlated to a phase of maximal synthetic activity of the nucleus. An interesting feature of the amphibian lampbrush stage oocyte nucleus is the immense number of nucleoli that may be present. The very large lampbrush chromosomes are subdivided linearly into chromomeres and inter-chromomeres and each chromosome consists of only two chromatids. In metabolically active growing oocytes, such as those found in amphibians, pairs of lateral loops develop from the chromomeres and it has been estimated that as many as 20,000 loops may be present in the *Triturus* lampbrush chromosomes. The size and structure of the loops that arise from most chromomeres is rather uniform although a few characteristically give rise to giant loops which show certain structural peculiarities. All loops have been shown to contain an axial element composed of DNA which is more or less surrounded by a matrix of ribonucleoprotein.

The studies of Gall and Callan (192) as well as those of Miller (360) and of Izawa et al. (258) have indicated that each loop represents an extended active genetic locus. Since the loops have been found to be centers of active RNA synthesis they are considered to be sites of intense gene activity. Callan (112) has found that the nucleolar organizer regions in the lampbrush stage bud off large numbers of DNA rings each of which forms a free nucleolus, thus amplifying by lavish means the flow of genetic information from a specific locus. The RNA present in the lampbrush stage of the *Triturus* oocyte was isolated and analyzed by Edström and Gall (168). In those studies the chromosomes, nucleoli, and nuclear sap were isolated separately and the nucleotide base composition of their RNA was determined. The results of those studies demonstrated that the chromosomal RNA was DNA-like in base composition while that of the nucleolus contained RNA of the ribosomal type. The RNA of the nuclear sap constituted most of the RNA of the nucleus and was essentially of an anomalous type.

Izawa et al. (257) demonstrated that the loops can be made to regress to a condensed state and stop synthesizing RNA by adding arginine-rich but not lysine-rich histone to the system. Similar results were obtained by treatment with actinomycin D.

One interesting aspect of lampbrush chromosome loops is their polar structure. Gall and Callan (192) demonstrated with the use of tritiated uridine that the polarity is a reflection of a polarity in function. In some of the largest loops studied it was found that the incorporation of uridine always begins at one initial section situated at one end of the loop. As time passed, the leading edge of the labeling moved slowly forward until after several days it reached the far end of the loop. These workers interpreted their results as being due to the continuous motion of the loop axis. It was assumed that there is a fixed point of synthesis through which the entire length of the DNA strand must pass while it is spun out into the loop. A similar back-spooling mechanism at the other end of the loop would keep the loop size constant. Beermann (45), on the other hand, has interpreted these results differently. He has suggested the possibility that chromomere loops in general consist of an initial segment active in transcription followed by partially redundant posterior segments which may serve as substrate in the packaging and thus stabilize the DNA-like RNA produced in that chromomere.

Studies on the lampbrush chromosomes indicate, then, that localized chromosome sites, presumably individual genes or clusters of genes, can exist on a chromosome in two reversible states. The active RNA-forming state is spun out into a loop, while the inactive state, during which RNA is not synthesized, is condensed and appears to be associated with the arginine-rich histone fraction.

Equally striking visible evidence for selective gene activation has been adduced from the giant polytene chromosomes found in certain tissues of Diptera. In *Drosophila* and in various midges the cells of certain organs may become very large and contain enormous chromosomes. These giant interphase chromosomes may attain a length of at least ten times and a cross section of up to 10,000 times that of normal univalent interphase chromosomes. They are polytene, consisting of thousands of strands as a result of repeated chromatid replication without mitotic contraction and separation. When appropriately stained these giant chromosomes show a pattern of many light and dark crossbands. With the use of cytogenetic methods the precise position of a considerable number of individual genes has been accurately determined on certain of the chromosomes. It has been found, moreover, that all of the major bands of the chromosomes can be recognized in all tissues in which there is a reasonably good development of polytene chromosomes (457). Thus, morphologically at least, there appear to be no differences in the structure of the same chromosomes found in different tissues and any differences, if in fact such do exist, must be on a rather minute scale.

Beermann (43) made a detailed study of the fine structure of the polytene chromosomes of several tissues found in the midge species *Chironomus tentans*. This investigator found that although in all tissues studied the same sequence of bands was present in the same chromosomes, individual bands showed characteristic appearances in different tissues. Particular bands, different ones for different tissues, were swollen into puffs. Thus it was found, for example, that certain bands were puffed in the rectum but were compact in other tissues, while other bands were puffed in the Malpighians and in the salivary gland but were compact in the rectum, and so on. It was clear, therefore, from these and many similar studies that different tissues within an organism have different puffing patterns. Experiments with labeled compounds demonstrated, moreover, that puffed regions of the polytene chromosomes, like the loops of the lampbrush chromosomes, are active centers of RNA synthesis, as evidenced by the rapid uptake and incorporation of tritiated uridine (391).

Beermann (44) presented most impressive evidence that a puff may represent a single gene locus. He (44) found that the production of a component in the saliva of *Chironomus* depended on the existence of a puff in a particular chromomere of one of the chromosomes. This chromomere was also found by cytogenetic studies to be the site of the gene concerned with the production of the same secretion component. A spontaneous recessive mutant was isolated which in the homozygous condition lacked both the secretion component and the puff. In heterozygotes the puff was found to be produced in a heterozygous fashion. In cells not forming the puff, i.e., those not producing the specific secretion component, no structural difference between the mutated and normal chromomere could be detected. This elegant one gene–one puff analysis demonstrates most clearly that activity of the secretion-determining gene is correlated with its puffed appearance while its inactivity is related to its appearance as a condensed band. It is clear, moreover, that the activity of this gene is involved with the differentiation of a cell into a secretory cell. The results of this study indicate in the strongest possible manner, then, that differential gene activity is correlated with cellular differentiation. Beermann has found, moreover, that between 10% and 20% of the chromomeres are in a puffed or active form in any one cell type at any one time, while the rest are in an inactive or condensed state.

One would, of course, like very much to know what makes genes become active and how it happens that they become functional only in particular cells and at a definite stage of development. Very little is known about this sort of thing in any organism. It has, nevertheless, been found that characteristic puff patterns can be modified by environmental conditions. The postembryonic development of insects is under the control of at least two hormones. The prothoracic gland hormone ecdysone induces molting, while the juvenile hormone of the corpora allata tends to keep the insect in its larval form.

It has now been found in several insect species that if ecdysone is administered before pupation would normally occur, the puff pattern changes rapidly to that characteristic of the pupation stage and molting then takes place (121). Clever (122) has noted, moreover, that definite patterns of localized puffs appear in a definite time sequence following administration of the molting hormone. It is as if this hormone directly or indirectly activated a few genes and as if the action of those genes derepressed other genes in a definite sequential series. The derepression of one gene may thus be dependent upon prior derepression of another gene or genes. It has been suggested that although the immediate stimulus might be a circulating hormone to which all cells are exposed, only those cells possessing the appropriate pattern of other derepressed genes will respond to the action of the hormone.

Clever has found, furthermore, that mere variations in the amounts of hormone administered or in the relative amounts of two hormones reaching a cell may bring about different puff patterns.

Clever (121) and Karlson (273) were the first to suggest that the hormone ecdysone exerts its effects by specifically and directly activating two chromomere loci 1-18-C and IV-2B in *Chironomus tentans*. Kroeger, on the other hand, interpreted his observations as showing that ecdysone acts by changing the K^+/Na^+ ratio in the cell and that it is by high K^+ concentrations that the prepupal puffing pattern is induced (298). Clever (122) points out, however, that high K^+ concentrations do not affect the ecdysone-sensitive loci in *Chironomus* and that, moreover, ecdysone is active even in the absence of K^+ ions.

The significance of the large chromosomal puffs in development has recently been brought into question by the studies of Goodman et al. (208). Using *Sciara* as the experimental test object, these workers reported that essentially normal development occurred without the appearance of puffs and without the intense synthesis of RNA at the chromosomal sites at which puffs ordinarily appear although RNA synthesis proceeded normally elsewhere in the chromosomes. Larval development without puffs was produced by feeding the larvae cortisone, a vertebrate hormone not normally found in insects. This appears, therefore, to be the first instance which has been reported to produce puff suppression and still permit normal development to proceed. This study suggests, then, that although the formation of large puffs with accompanying RNA synthesis may serve as a convenient marker for the activity of certain genes, puffing does not appear to be essential for gene action, at least not in *Sciara*.

It should be mentioned, however, that results very recently obtained by Crouse (134a) are at variance with those reported by Goodman et al. (208). Different results were also reported by Smith et al. (463), who treated *Drosophila* with cortisone at a concentration of 10 mg/ml of medium and found that viability was reduced and development was largely inhibited. However, at concentrations of cortisone which permitted development to proceed, the puff patterns found were of the characteristic type. Since results reported in both studies are not in accord with those of Goodman et al., it seems wise to postpone further speculation regarding structure-function relationships in the regulation of gene activity in chromosomes until these matters are clarified.

Hormonal Activation of Genes. In addition to ecdysone, which is a steroid hormone, other steroid hormones appear clearly to be involved in the activation of genes. This is particularly well illustrated in the case of the estrogens. It has been found by many workers in many laboratories that if the ovaries are removed from an experimental animal and estrogen is administered, the synthesis of protein by cells of the uterus increases as much as 300% two to four hours after estrogen treatment. That this increase has to do with the synthesis of new protein is evidenced by the fact that the stimulating effects of estrogen are blocked by puromycin which specifically inhibits new protein synthesis. It has been found, moreover, that less than thirty minutes after hormone treatment there is a dramatic increase in the rate of RNA synthesis. When the antibiotic actinomycin D is used to block RNA synthesis, estrogen has no effect on protein synthesis. These studies suggest, then, that treatment of uterine cells with estrogenic hormones results in activation at the gene level and that this accounts for many of the diverse metabolic changes observed in such cells. These metabolic changes involve an increased synthesis of amino acids from glucose, the increased evolution of carbon dioxide, and an increased synthesis of lipids and phospholipids.

It is clear, moreover, that a significant number of genes must be activated in order to account for the many different responses observed in uterine cells treated with estrogen. If now, instead of treating uterine cells with estrogen, one treats liver cells, an entirely different result is obtained. It is well known that when an egg is being formed in a hen, the estrogen produced by the hen's ovaries stimulates its liver to produce two yolk proteins, phosvitin and lipovitellin. These proteins are not normally synthesized by a rooster. However, if estrogen is administered to a rooster, its liver will produce large amounts of these egg yolk proteins. It would be difficult, indeed, to find a more striking instance of the selective activation of repressed genes than is provided by the above example. The gene-activating effect of estrogen appears, moreover, to be highly specific. Phosvitin is an unusual protein in that almost one-half of its amino acid residues are of one kind, serine. Carlsen et al. (113) have found that estrogen causes liver cells to synthesize large amounts of a species of transfer RNA that is concerned specifically with the incorporation of serine into protein.

Thus, the effect of estrogen on uterine cells is quite different from its effect on liver cells although in both instances different genes in the two cell types appear to be selectively derepressd and, hence, rendered functional. It may be suggested, therefore, that hormonal specificity resides both in the hormone itself and in the protoplasmic substrate upon which the hormone acts in a target cell. There is evidence, furthermore, that other steroid hormones such as testosterone, aldosterone, and cortisone exert their effects, in part at least, through activation of genes. Even such nonsteroid hormones as thyroxin and insulin may operate, in part at least, via gene activation. This is suggested by the studies of Kidson and Kirby (281) who injected these and certain other hormones into rats and measured the synthesis of DNA-like RNA. The most striking aspect of those studies was the extremely short time lag, which amounted to about fifteen minutes, between administration of the hormone and the change in pattern of RNA synthesis. In these instances the synthesis of new RNA in the affected cells occurred in so short a period of time that the results obtained would suggest that gene activation may be the initial site of hormone action.

All of these studies raise the much more fundamental questions as to precisely how genes are selectively activated by a given hormone, whether such genes are, in fact, preset for hormonal activation in target cells and, finally, how the hormone interacts not only with the gene itself but with the entire system of genetic regulation. The evidence presented until now goes only as far as to show that an early stage in the operation of a number of hormones is the selective stimulation of genetic activity in a target cell. This entire matter was considered by Eric H. Davidson in *Scientific American* in 1965.

Activation of Genes by the Cytoplasm. That nucleocytoplasmic exchange is a primary interaction in the developmental reading of the genome is clearly indicated in many of the now classical embryological studies. For example, certain sea urchin eggs are clear spherules which contain a broad band of cytoplasmic pigment granules that can be used as a marker to orient the egg. If an unfertilized egg is cut into halves parallel to but just above the pigment band, the halves will round up and heal. If each half is now fertilized by a sperm, both halves will cleave and the upper or animal half without the pigment band develops into a blastula (dauerblastula) but fails to form endoderm. The lower or vegetal half with the pigment band, on the other hand, develops into an incomplete embryo. A very different result is obtained, however, if an unfertilized egg is cut perpendicular to the pigment band. On fertilization, each half produces a larva that is complete but somewhat reduced in size. It is clear, therefore, that everything necessary to produce the complete larva is contained in half the egg when it is cut perpendicular to the pigment band but not when cut parallel to it.

From findings such as these it is possible to draw two main conclusions. First, the cytoplasm of the egg cell is not homogeneous and cytoplasmic materials required for development are localized to a significant extent. Normal development proceeds only in that part that contains at least a portion or all of the specific cytoplasmic components. Second, equivalent sperm nuclei introduced into each of three (upper, lower, or lateral) halves function in three different kinds of development. Thus the assumption can be made that the behavior of the nucleus is not programmed entirely internally but rather that its activity must depend, in part at least, upon the nature of the cytoplasm in which it resides (215).

Similar results have been obtained with amphibian eggs. The essential structure of such eggs at the time of fertilization is quite simple. Yolk platelets tend to concentrate at the lower or vegetative pole while the nucleus is commonly found at the other or animal end. Soon after fertilization a further regional difference appears. A special cytoplasmic region known as the "gray crescent" appears slightly below the equator of the egg and is concentrated on one side of the main axis. This special cytoplasmic region plays an extremely important role all through early development. The importance of the gray crescent for future development was established many years ago. If, for example, a newt's egg is pinched into two, both halves will produce a complete normal adult. If, on the other hand, the plane of constriction is such that the entire crescent is present in one half, the second half may undergo cell division if it contains a nucleus but it never produces any of the characteristic features of adult tissues. Its cells remain embryonic and without a capacity for specific differentiation. It thus appears that it is the crescent-containing cytoplasm that first switches on the gene activities that control the synthesis of proteins concerned with differentiated function. Cells free of gray crescent material can presumably synthesize proteins required for the mitotic apparatus but they do not seem to be able to synthesize other types of specialized proteins (534).

These and numerous other classical studies have thus provided a theoretical orientation with which to approach the problem of selective gene activation during early embryogenesis. It is now possible, moreover, to study selective gene activity in concrete terms by measuring the synthesis of the specific gene product mRNA and thus to examine directly the proposition that the egg cytoplasm contains substances capable of functioning directly or indirectly as selective activators of the cellular genome.

An interesting example to illustrate this type of approach (and this is just one of several that could be cited) deals with the early development of the gastropod mollusk *Ilyanassa obsoleta*. In *Ilyanassa*, a region of the egg cytoplasm known as the "polar lobe" is transiently extruded as a spherical lobe several times during maturation and early cleavage divisions. If this lobe is removed, the embryos continue to develop as free-swimming motile forms containing muscle, velar cilia, enteron, stromodium, and digestive-gland tissue. They lack, however, the ability to produce certain characteristic tissues. Thus, stored exclusively in the polar lobe cytoplasm are substances needed for normal activation of cells inheriting that cytoplasm. Studies by Clement (118, 119, 120) have shown that the polar lobe of *Ilyanassa* contains cytoplasmic factors necessary for the production of intestine, heart, shell gland, as well as major mesodermal derivatives responsible for later structural organization.

In this species organ differentiation is well under way by the fourth day of development and from that time on the rate of bulk RNA accumulation is about the same in normal and lobeless embryos. Davidson et al. (141) studied RNA synthesis by lobeless and normal embryos during early stages of development. During the initial period of development no quantitative differences in the RNA synthesis of lobeless and normal embryos could be detected, but as development proceeded normal embryos displayed considerably more activity than did lobeless embryos. It is a few hours after gastrulation, in contrast to what is found in *Xenopus* (95), that a major increase in RNA synthesis becomes evident. It is at that point in development that lobeless and normal embryos show a 1.5 to twofold difference in RNA synthesis. During this period of development ribosomal RNA synthesis probably constitutes only a negligible fraction of the observed RNA synthesis since Collier (125) has demonstrated that bulk RNA content does not begin to increase until the fourth day of development. The difference in RNA synthesis observed in the lobeless and normal embryos has been interpreted by Davidson et al. (141) to represent a difference in the level of gene activation in the two types of embryos.

Localization of cytoplasmic factors that are later involved in selective gene activation appears to be a general phenomenon. Such gene activating factors have been demonstrated to exist in egg cytoplasm not only of molluscan forms but also in amphibians (177, 136), annelids (381), ascidians (129), insects (234, 254), and echinoderms (157), as well as in other groups of animals. An elucidation of the mechanism by which such prelocalized cytoplasmic factors affect the activity of embryonic nuclei would clearly constitute an explanation for differentiation in early development. For purposes of this discussion, however, it is sufficient to note that selective gene activation is mediated in early embryogenesis by cytoplasmically localized substances.

Two additional fundamental concepts of development, that of induction leading to determination and that of cellular competence, should be considered. The thoughts presented here concerning these matters are those recently expressed by Wolff (567a).

Induction Leading to Determination and Differentiation. Following the discovery of the "organization center" in the amphibian embryo by Spemann (474) and of its inductive action on the overlying ectodermal layer leading to the development of the neural plate (475), a very large number of studies have been focused on the phenomenon of embryonic induction since, as is now recognized, it represents one of the basic mechanisms in morphogenesis. It is now clear that the whole of development may be explained by a series of inductions in which each anlage successively acts as an inductor of a still undetermined anlage. In the amphibian egg the first determination takes place in the chordamesoderm anlage which acts as the primary inductor of the nervous system. From that point onward the whole of organogenesis is an uninterrupted sequence of inductions. It has thus now been clearly demonstrated that most differentiations are determined by inductors and that many operate at a distance, as was first demonstrated by Niu and Twitty (378). Similarly, inductors of certain special structures may exert their effects through artificial membranes as evidenced by the inducing action of the ureter on metanephric mesenchyme in mammals (214) and birds (111). These studies point to the probability of specific substances being involved.

What, then, is the nature of such substances? The first example of a known substance acting as an inductor of an embryonic structure at a late stage in organogenesis was the finding of Wolff and Ginglinger (568) that steroid hormones controlled the differentiation of gonads. While it is not as yet known whether steroid hormones are the natural inductors, they, nevertheless, have the same effects. More recently some information on the nature of inductors concerned with the primary organization of the amphibian egg has been obtained. For example, Toivonen (520, 521), Tiedemann (514), and Yamada (575) succeeded in isolating two groups of proteins with distinct chemical and biological properties. One of these, a mesodermal inductor, is unstable and very sensitive to high temperatures. It has the specific property of inducing chorda, muscle, connective tissue, etc. A second protein, which is a nucleoprotein and is associated with RNA, has a neuralizing effect and, more particularly, possesses the capacity of inducing the anterior brain in presumptive ectoderm.

When both of these inductors are placed together *in vitro* between two sheets of presumptive ectoderm many of the structures of a normal embryo are induced. According to Toivonen et al. (521) both substances are localized in the normal embryo in two inverse gradients. One of these is oriented in the caudocephalic direction, the other in the cephalocaudal direction. According to Tiedemann and Tiedemann (515), if the ratio of neuralizing protein to mesodermalizing factor is 50 to 1, the differentiation of cerebral structures, particularly the telecephalon, will be induced. If that ratio is reduced to 10 to 1, deuterencephalic organs will differentiate, while if the proportions are reduced to 1 to 1, only trunk-caudal differentiations are induced. It is indeed quite remarkable that undetermined ectoderm, which by itself is unable to differentiate, can be made to differentiate into numerous highly complex structures under the influence of special and presumably specific proteins.

This, then, raises the question as to whether inductors do, in fact, possess specificity as appears to be the case in the results reported above, or whether, as is commonly believed, the specificity resides within the competent cell. The studies of Baltzer (27) bear on this question. This investigator demonstrated that the same inductor which determines the formation of balancers in urodeles determines the formation of suckers in anurans. These studies indicate, then, that competent cells respond according to their specific potentialities and yet, since it is an adhesive organ that is formed in both cases, the inductor must also possess a certain specificity. It is, moreover, not unlikely that inductors are generally specific substances and in most instances in the animal field appear to be proteins or nucleoproteins. Yet, one cannot ignore the older extensive literature dealing with "nonspecific" induction effects in which, as in the case of oncogenesis, substances of the most diverse type were found to act as effective inductors. The studies of Barth (38) have shown, moreover, that ions will induce various cell types from the presumptive epidermis of the *Rana pipiens* gastrula.

In plants, on the other hand, development appears to be controlled in part at least by two main groups of morphogenetic substances, the auxins and the cytokinins. By varying the ratio of these two substances in an otherwise suitable culture medium and with the use of competent cells, it is possible to induce the formation of most organs of a plant, at least under *in vitro* conditions (see Fig. 8) (456). Just how these biologically active substances exert their effects is not known. The evidence thus far available does not preclude the possibility that they act indirectly by stimulating or inhibiting true inductors which would be specific substances involved in the induction of roots, leaves, flowers, etc.

The Competence Concept. An inductive action must obviously represent an interaction between an inducing system and a reacting system. The inducing system produces an inductive agent while the reacting system must at the same time be able to respond to it. This reactivity has been called competence by Waddington (534). The mechanisms underlying cellular competence have not in the past been subject to a great deal of experimental study. It is a rather difficult problem to analyze experimentally. It is, nevertheless, well known that presumptive ectoderm (neuro-epidermis) is multicompetent in that it may develop in any one or more of several different directions depending on the inductors that it encounters in the embryo or to which it may be subjected experimentally. It may, for example, differentiate into basal epidermis and give rise to scales in reptiles, feathers in birds, and hair, nails, and tooth enamel in mammals. Under different

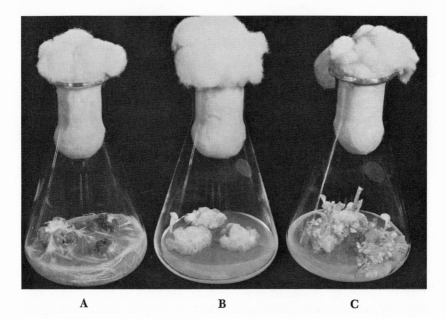

A   **B**   **C**

Fig. 8. The effect of the ratio of two plant growth-regulating substances, the auxins (indoleacetic acid) and the cytokinins (kinetin), on the growth patterns of normal tobacco tissue in culture. All flasks contained 2 mg/l of indoleacetic acid in a modified White's basic culture medium. In addition, flask **A** contained 0.02 mg/l of kinetin; note extensive development of roots. Flask **B** contained 0.2 mg/l of kinetin; the tissues in this instance grew in an essentially unorganized manner. Flask **C** contained 0.5 mg/l of kinetin; under those conditions of culture a profusion of shoots developed. (Courtesy of Dr. Folke Skoog.)

environmental conditions it can develop into pigment cells, while in other situations it will differentiate into any part of the nervous system.

These potentialities for differentiation in different directions may, however, gradually be lost either through aging or through treatment with X rays. Several authors (117, 193, 242, 375) have studied neural competence of the ectoderm and have found that the reacting system during its normal aging process passes through successive periods of competence for different inductive actions. Similarly, Reyss-Brion (412, 413) has found that when presumptive ectoderm is isolated, placed in culture, and treated with increasing doses of X rays, it progressively loses a capacity to develop the different neural structures under the influence of primary inductors. The capacity for developing deuterencephalic structures is lost first, then the ability to form archencephalic structures disappears, while the last to remain is the capacity to form spinocaudal structures. Presumptive ectoderm is, moreover, unable to differentiate into any organized structure when irradiation doses of more than 1,000 R are administered. It is thus possible to dissociate experimentally several potentialities of an undetermined tissue and, hence, to begin to analyze competence in a system such as that described above.

We still know very little about the biochemical nature of competence although the suggestion of Flickinger and Stone (181) that competence may be characterized by the presence of specific antigens should be mentioned here.

It is tempting to speculate that gene activation by inducing substances is similar to the action of hormones described earlier except that induction gives rise to stable cellular changes. If that is true, the competence of a cell would merely reflect an appropriate pattern of other derepressed genes just as has been postulated for the target cell of a hormone.

The Stability of the Differentiated State. The term differentiation is commonly used to describe the more stable cellular changes that occur during the development of a plant or animal. A distinction is often drawn between such stable changes and modulations (545) which are by definition more readily reversible. It is, nevertheless, clear that from whatever level one looks at differentiation, one sees a continuously graded series ranging from the most stable and apparently irreversible, on the one hand, to the most transient, on the other. Sonneborn (467) has pointed out, moreover, that exactly the same cellular traits that appear to be highly stable and even irreversible in some cell types are readily reversible or alterable in other cell types. It is not, therefore, the change that varies in such instances but rather the associated mechanisms which result either in its stable fixation or in its modifiability. The distinction between differentiation and modulation as ordinarily defined is not, therefore, easy to preserve, especially in view of what is now known about cell behavior during regeneration.

Perhaps the clearest examples of cells which have attained an irreversibly differentiated state include among others the mature red blood cells of mammals and the lens fiber cells, both of which have lost their nuclei. These are, however, very special cases and represent extreme examples of terminal differentiation. The differentiation process in certain nucleated cells such as, for example, the mature nerve cell is highly stable and may well be irreversible. It is, however, possible to influence experimentally cellular differentiation in many ways. One of the best known of these is the effect of the thiocyanate and lithium ions on embryonic development. The former switches differentiation toward the ectoderm (animalization), the latter toward the endoderm (vegetalization). An interesting example of an experimentally induced metaplasia, the change of character of one cell type to another, was reported by Fell and Mellanby (178). Explants of chick ectoderm normally differentiate into a squamous keratinized epithelium. These workers found, however, that if treated with an excess of vitamin A, such cells can be made to switch their pattern of differentiation and develop into ciliated mucous-secreting cells. When the exogenous source of vitamin A is removed, the normal pattern of differentiation is resumed. Since no transformation of cornifying cells to mucous-secreting cells or vice versa was recorded in these studies, the plasticity of the cells of the ectoderm lies in the presence of immature cells which respond to the vitamin and not in the plasticity of the fully differentiated cells.

Weiss and James (547) confirmed those experiments and demonstrated that treatment with vitamin A for as short a period as fifteen minutes is sufficient to produce the switch in differentiation. This sort of thing is, moreover, not uncommon in the lower forms. Willmer (561) found that the protozoan *Naegleria gruberi* can be made to grow either as an amoeboid or as a flagellate form by manipulating the ionic environment to which the organism is exposed. Examples of metaplasia are commonly found in the literature of pathology. Willis (559), for example, describes the appearance of bone in adenocarcinomas of the stomach or prostate as well as in old inflammatory foci or the occurrence of striated muscle in mixed tumors of the endometrium. On the basis of these and many other similar examples Willis (560) states:

The student of normal histology is apt to assume that the different kinds of adult tissues and cells are rigidly fixed invariable structures, distinct immutable species each capable of producing by proliferation cells of the one kind only. But, as soon as he pays attention to pathological histology—that is, to what the various cells and tissues can be and do in all manner of abnormal environments—he realizes that great transformations of cellular structure are possible in most tissues. The cells have much wider potencies for differentiation than are ever displayed in health; abnormal conditions are needed to reveal their dormant potencies or plasticity.

It is doubtless true, as Grobstein has suggested (215), that intensive study of metaplasia in normal systems has been delayed by the deterministic assumption that Willis refers to above.

Perhaps the most conclusive evidence for the occurrence of true metaplasia comes from the rather special but now well-documented case of the so-called Wolffian regeneration of the lens. If the lens is removed from the eye of a salamander, the differentiated iris epithelial cells lose their pigment, dedifferentiate, and undergo proliferation to form a spherical mass from which they transform into differentiated lens cells and ultimately into lens fibers (411). The iris epithelial cells need not suffer wounding in order to regenerate. Evidence has now accumulated in support of the idea that the factor involved in the transformation of the iris into lens depends on the retina. Complete suppression of lens regeneration can be achieved by removing neural retina, pigmented retina, and choroid together with lens. Under those conditions no regeneration of the neural retina occurs (494) and lens regeneration is suppressed. It has also been found that in the lentectomized eye, the separation of the dorsal iris from the retina by a piece of pliofilm prevents transformation of the dorsal iris into lens (492, 493).

The fact that iris epithelial cells synthesize tissue-specific antigens and melanin granules (332) and are arranged as a specific epithelium suggesting specific cell affinity indicates that the iris epithelium is a specific tissue which is regularly capable, under suitable conditions, of dedifferentiating and redifferentiating into a new direction.

Stone (490, 491) has described in detail cellular metaplasia involving derivatives of epithelial origin in which the regeneration of sensory retina from pigmented epithelium or tapetum of adult salamander eyes occurred. Thus, in this instance progeny of pigment-forming cells lost this characteristic property and developed into highly differentiated neural cells of the retina.

Coulombre and Coulombre (131) in an elegant inversion experiment found that when the lens of a five-day chick embryo was reversed by surgical procedure so that the internal side of the lens came to face the cornea and the original external side faced the retina, the lens epithelium was transformed into fiber cells. Some factor or condition must, therefore, be operative in the posterior chamber of the eye which transforms epithelial cells into fiber cells.

There are other situations in which at least some differentiated cells can be caused to lose their initial differentiation and then develop along entirely different pathways. This is certainly true of somatic cells of certain plant species as well as those found in certain lower animals where the differentiated state does not appear to be as strongly determined and hence as stable as it is in mammals. However, a large number of different transformations have been reported between certain classically accepted but relatively unspecialized cell types or from relatively unspecialized to specialized cell types in mammals. The origin of macrophages not only from muscle elements (116) but from epithelial (116) and Schwann cells (546, 548) are examples of this type. Politzer (398) and McCreight and Andrew (349) have reported on the interconversion of epithelial and mes-enchymally derived tissues in postfetal stages and even in the adult. Mesenchyme appears, moreover, normally to transform into epithelial in the kidneys. The appearance of bone in rabbit muscle as described by Levander (304) appears to be an example of tissue metaplasia. There seem, however, to be no well-documented examples of the direct conversion of one highly specialized cell type into another in mammals (215).

Interesting examples of metaplasia are found in such vertebrates as newts and salamanders that possess pronounced capacities to restore by regeneration lost or injured parts. In these instances when a limb or a tail is removed, the first evidence for regeneration is the accumulation at the wound surface of a small bundle of embryonic-appearing cells known as the blastema. It had long been argued by some that in animals that can regenerate, the body contains a reserve supply of embryonic cells scattered among the tissues and it is those cells that accumulate at the wound site to form the blastema, which then begins to develop and differentiate to restore the injured or lost part. However, certain types of experiments have raised doubts concerning the correctness of that interpretation (535). It is known that if animals are subjected to X-irradiation, even if the treatment is carried out some months before amputation of a limb, regeneration is stopped entirely. If, for example, a forelimb of an X-ray-treated animal is removed and enough time is allowed to elapse to be certain that regeneration will not occur, after which the limb from an unirradiated newt is grafted onto the stump, the grafted limb will heal in a satisfactory manner. If, now, the grafted limb is, in turn, amputated leaving only a small disc of unirradiated tissue attached to the stump of the X-rayed animal, regeneration occurs. This appears to be very good evidence that the cells of the blastema which develop into a new limb are derived locally. The evidence appears to indicate, moreover, that muscle cells and perhaps other cell types such as cartilage and Schwann cells at the wound site dedifferentiate and then constitute the blastema from which regeneration occurs (232a).

It has been shown, furthermore, that if the humerus is removed from a newt forelimb, it is not regenerated. If, now, this boneless arm is amputated, a regenerate grows out of the stump and does contain a new humerus although no normal bone-forming cells were present at the cut surface. Findings such as these appear to demonstrate, then, that the cells that form the blastema do return, to some extent at least, to the embryonic condition and are quite capable of differentiating again along new and different pathways. However, the cells of the blastema do not appear to have become fully embryonic since attempts to cause blastema produced on stumps of amputated tails to develop limbs, and vice versa, have as yet met with little success.

The evidence provided by histological metaplasia is of great importance for an understanding of the problem of determination which, as defined by Hadorn (222), is "a process which initiates a specific pathway of development by singling it out from among various possibilities for which a cellular system is competent." The evidence presented above demonstrates, among other things, that the determination which occurs in embryonic stages and the high degree of histological differentiation which follows it need not necessarily involve irreversible changes despite the fact that shortly after the period of embryonic determination in vertebrates the resulting cellular differentiation appears to be highly stable. Yet, if the experiments on regeneration described above have been interpreted correctly, it is obvious that much later in life the stimulus of wounding may have precisely the effect of bringing mature determined cells back to a more plastic condition from which they can again differentiate in any one or more of several new directions. It therefore follows that the nuclear genes which are involved in the differentiation of new histological types must have persisted throughout development in the previously determined cells. Whether the entire genotype is conserved remains a matter of conjecture since we do not as yet know the full range of potentialities of blastema cells.

Determination and Transdetermination. Further significant investigations on the stability of the differentiated state following determination come from the studies of Hadorn and his associates (222). These investigators have studied cultures of determined cell populations that were derived from imaginal discs of *Drosophila* larvae. Experiments which were carried out with the use of male or female genital discs or antennae or leg discs have led to similar conclusions. The male genital disc, for example, contains not only the anlagen for the internal sex organs but also forms the external genitalia and the anal plate with the hindgut. In the third larval instar this disc consists of small densely packed cells which are all very similar in appearance and show no evidence of specific differentiation. It has been established by a number of different methods (223, 380, 524), however, that all of the cells of the disc are specifically determined. A genital disc thus contains a mosaic of blastemas and the cells of each blastema are determined for forming just one of the several elements which comprise the genital apparatus.

Determined cells of larval discs were cultured in abdomens of adult flies where they continued to divide profusely, being transferred to new adults every 2 weeks for a period of up to 3 years. In the abdomen of the adult, cells of such cultures maintain their essentially undifferentiated larval characteristics. When, however, such cells are reimplanted into larvae, the cells undergo metamorphosis to form normal adult organs, indicating that the initial determined state may be conserved in the dividing cells for periods up to 3 years. In addition, cell lines have been obtained from cultivated disc primordia which no longer differentiate into genital organs. These were found to switch into other states of determination which resulted in the differentiation of antennae, legs, wings, and thorax. Such trans-determinations occur regularly and with reproducible probability. Certain sequences can thus be followed. From anal plate blastemas, primordia of antennae and legs arise first. Then, in a second trans-ducing step, the characteristics for wing structures are established, and finally the descendants of wing cells are often transdetermined into thorax blastemas.

It is clear from these studies that the *in vivo* cultures of imaginal discs provide a most favorable material for maintaining proliferating cells for long periods of time in a determined or programmed state such that they will not undergo adult differentiation. Thus, in this system the process of determination can be sharply separated from later steps of differentiation. There is, moreover, considerable evidence that determination is carried by individual cells rather than by the organ anlagen as a whole. It has been shown, moreover, that changes in determination occur in clones derived from determined cells. This leads to a new type of determination which can again be propagated or which may undergo further change. The evidence suggests that cell divisions are a necessary prerequisite for transdetermination. Since transdetermination is a directed and reversible process which presumably occurs in groups of adjoining cells simultaneously, it is assumed that it involves changes in gene activity rather than changes in the integrity of the genetic material. Although the mechanism underlying determination is not at present understood, it certainly does not appear to be based on any irreversible nuclear or cytoplasmic change. This is an unusually favorable material for studying the very fundamental problem of determination, and it may ultimately provide the key to the whole problem of cell differentiation.

There seems, then, to be rather good evidence that differentiation along certain pathways at least can under certain circumstances be reversed. However, it is usually not easy to reverse the differentiated state and it is only in a few relatively favorable instances that success has, as yet, been achieved. This does not, of course, mean that in the vast majority of instances in which reversibility has not been demonstrable that those cells are necessarily irreversibly differentiated. It probably means that we do not as yet know how to reverse the differentiated state in most instances. This is particularly true, as pointed out earlier, when one considers that exactly the same cellular traits that appear to be highly stable and perhaps even irreversible in some cell types are readily reversible or at least modifiable in other cell types. It would appear more probable that cell differentiation is, in all but certain select instances, a potentially reversible process. These thoughts should be kept in mind when the reversal of the tumorous state is discussed in Chapter VI.

Anomalous Differentiation and Development. When breakdowns in the processes involved in normal development occur, almost every conceivable developmental anomaly may result. However, only a limited portion of the very extensive subject of teratology is of interest to the oncologist. Schwalbe (447), in his elaborate treatise on that subject, has emphasized the existence of a continuous series from identical twins, to conjoined twins, through double monsters, parasitic fetuses (epignathi), teratomas, and mixed tumors down to more characteristic tumors that may be either benign or malignant (see Fig. 9). Before continuing this discussion it would be appropriate to describe briefly the growth phenomena that we are considering.

Teratological studies have now defined the origin of identical twins and conjoined twins and have greatly narrowed the range of possibilities for the development of most double monsters. The parasitic fetus appears to be attributable in origin either to a second embryo which in some way becomes attached to the tissues of its host or, more commonly, to a process of budding, especially in those instances in which the parasitic growths are multiple and their development markedly imperfect. These remarkable developmental anomalies are congenital and are usually encountered in deformed stillborn fetuses. They may protrude from the pharynx or originate in the sacral region or in the thoracic or abdominal cavities. The parasitic fetus is characterized by growths that often present unmistakable parts of a fetus. In some instances the main tumor consists of a rudimentary head with or without brain tissue and well-formed organs as well as extremities with fingers, toes, and nails, all of which are present in

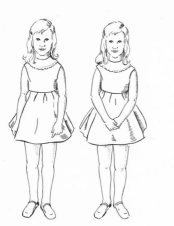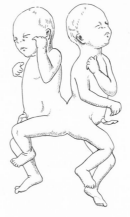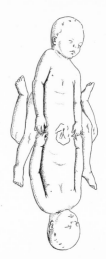

Identical twins.   Conjoined twins.   Double monsters.

Fig. 9. Investigations have disclosed a continuous spectrum which progresses from identical twins at the one end to cancers at the other. All that distinguishes the various abnormalities, one from another, is the stage in development at which the mishap occurs. Two daughter cells produced by the first division of the fertilized ovum, if their accidental separation is complete, give rise to normal identical twins. If the two cells are but partially separated, the outcome depends not only on the degree of attachment but also on the degree of development that

more or less orderly arrangement giving the appearance of a rudimentary fetus.

These growths differ from the teratomas, which represent the next stage in Schwalbe's series, in that the teratoma shows a complete or almost complete absence of organization of its often well-differentiated cells and tissues into a whole, although isolated morphological forms such as teeth found in teratomas may be very complete. The teratoma is not, then, a distorted fetus. It is characterized rather by chaotic tissue formation and, according to Willis (560), contains no true somatic regions. There are, in other words, masses of nerve tissue but no brain, renal tissue but no kidney, and bone tissue but no bones. It is interesting to note that despite chaotic distribution, the tissues found in the teratoma may be functional. Thus, teratomatous muscle may contract and the sweat glands, hemopoietic red marrow, and choroid plexus may secrete and perform essentially normal functions.

According to Willis (558), ovarian teratomas are often benign while those that arise in the testes are frequently malignant. When an ovarian teratoma becomes malignant, only one component of the

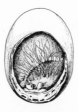

Ovarian dermoid teratoma (benign).

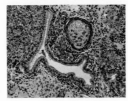

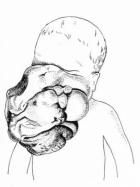

Conventional
tumors
(benign and
malignant).

Parasitic fetus
(epignathus).

Section of teratocarcinoma
(malignant).

each member of the pair undergoes. Thus, the result may be conjoined twins, double monsters, or a parasitic fetus. The benign and malignant teratomas arise from undetermined cells and are able to form many of the body tissues but are not capable of giving rise to an embryo, however primitive that may be. The conventional tumors develop from cells that have been determined and, hence, are commonly composed of a single cell type. (The illustration of a section of a malignant teratocarcinoma was kindly supplied by Dr. G. Barry Pierce, Jr.)

tumor is generally affected. Thus, if an epidermal cell becomes cancerous, a squamous cell carcinoma quite similar to any other epidermal carcinoma is produced. In the case of malignant teratomas of testicular origin, on the other hand, metastasis may frequently exhibit many of the differentiated derivatives that are found in the primary growth. This is understandable in the light of results reported by Kleinsmith and Pierce (292) dealing with a malignant testicular teratocarcinoma of the mouse which will be considered in detail in Chapter VI. It is sufficient to indicate here that the malignant component of this tumor was found to be a multipotential and essentially undifferentiated cell, the embryonal carcinoma cell, that was capable of giving rise to as many as fourteen distinct differentiated derivatives which together with the embryonal carcinoma cell represented all of the components found in the initial tumor.

Teratoma-like structures have been produced experimentally in a number of different ways. For example, Michalowsky (356) and, later, Bagg (25) have induced transplantable teratomata by injecting 5% zinc chloride into the testes of fowl. These experimentally induced teratomas may contain cartilage, bone, nerve tissue, muscle, fat, connective tissue, glands, epithelium, and carcinomatous or adeno-carcinomatous tissue. Needham (371) believes that what lies behind the growth anomalies such as those found in teratomas is the failure of an individuation field to control the action of evocating substances.

In a number of interesting researches Witschi (563, 564, 565, 566) has confirmed experimentally, in large part at least, Schwalbe's suggestion of the existence of an unbroken series of developmental anomalies that range from double monsters to malignant tumors. These studies have been reviewed by Witschi (567). This investigator fertilized with sperm frog eggs in various stages of overripeness and obtained most interesting results. When, for example, the eggs were kept for a relatively short period of time before fertilization, abnormal sex ratios were found which under the best conditions resulted in the production of 90% males. Those eggs that were kept somewhat longer before fertilization gave rise to significant numbers of double monsters, while those kept still longer developed teratomatous pro-liferations. When overripeness proceeded still further before fertiliza-tion, large tumorous masses appeared in the endoderm and epithe-liomas in the ectoderm of some of the otherwise highly abnormal embryos. Witschi transplanted cells from such tumorous growths into frogs and found that they not only established themselves and grew in an expanding manner but also penetrated the bladder and destroyed it and metastasized into the liver.

Embryonic abnormalities appear to be of fairly common occurrence following fertilization of overripe eggs, as evidenced by the studies of Blandau and Young (61) on guinea pig eggs and Lillie's work (308) on annelid development.

Studies of the type described above indicate that what primarily distinguishes the various growth abnormalities one from another is the stage at which the developmental mishap occurs. They suggest in the strongest possible manner, moreover, that the tumor problem generally is basically an extreme aspect of the problem of develop-ment. If that concept is correct, then the factors that regulate normal growth and development should also apply to the tumor problem. It should thus be possible in certain of the more favorable situations to reverse the neoplastic state just as it is now possible in certain instances to change the differentiated state of a normal cell. More importantly, however, we have in the concept of active and inactive gene states within a constant cellular genome a very real and, above all, an experimentally testable alternative to the concept of somatic cell mutation as an explanation for the heritable cellular change that underlies the tumorous state generally.

CHAPTER VI

Reversal of Tumor Growth

Since the concept of irreversibility of the tumorous state has over the years so completely dominated the thinking of experimental oncologists very little basic research was carried out until quite recently to determine whether it might, in fact, be possible to cause a malignant cell to revert to the nonmalignant state. It should be emphasized at this point that reversion to the nonmalignant state need not necessarily mean reversion to the normal state. It will be recalled that many secondary changes such as, for example, aneuploidy, alterations in respiration, the deletion of enzymes, etc., may and do occur quite commonly in certain tumors. Thus, even if those properties of a cell that lead to autonomous growth were potentially reversible, the result would not necessarily be a completely normal cell since the recovered cell might retain the secondarily acquired properties originally possessed by the tumor cell. Even though such a reverted cell would be abnormal it would, nevertheless, be benign and, hence, fulfill the criteria for the reversion from the malignant to the nonmalignant state.

The unequivocal demonstration of the conversion of truly autonomous tumor cells into normal cells under defined experimental conditions could have great conceptual implications, since it would provide the ultimate proof that the malignant state may be mediated through purely epigenetic mechanisms. Implicit in that thought rests the concept that stable phenotypes can arise in somatic cells without concomitant changes in the integrity of the genetic determinants that are normally present in a cell. More importantly, such a concept would imply that the neoplastic transformation generally may be a potentially reversible process and, if that is true, could, theoretically at least, provide entirely new avenues of approach to cancer therapy. That a reversal of the neoplastic state may, in fact, occur has now been well documented in a wide spectrum of organisms ranging from higher plant species to man. Selected examples of a type that best illustrate this phenomenon are described below.

Reversal of the Tumorous State in Plants

The Crown Gall Disease

The first successful attempts to convert autonomous and transplantable tumor cells into normal or at least mature differentiated cell types under controlled experimental conditions were those carried out with the use of plant tumor systems as experimental models. Of these the non-self-limiting neoplastic disease of plants commonly known as crown gall has been most thoroughly investigated. As indicated earlier, the typical crown gall tumor cell appears to be an irreversibly altered cell. Such cell types isolated from many different plant species have been maintained in culture for periods up to two decades without showing the slightest tendency to become less autonomous. These tumor cells are transplantable. They are, therefore, persistently altered cells that reproduce true to type and against the growth of which there are no adequate control mechanisms in a host.

In studying the origin of the crown gall tumor cell attempts were made to distinguish between somatic mutation at the nuclear gene level, involving the deletion or permanent rearrangement of genetic information, on the one hand, and epigenetic changes which are concerned merely with alterations in the expression of the genetic potentialities that are normally present in a cell, on the other. It is unfortunately not possible to carry out breeding experiments of the classical type in this and similar systems and thus determine whether segregation of a possible mutation occurs at meiosis according to the Mendelian laws of heredity. Other less direct methods had, therefore, to be applied.

For studies of this type plants offer at least two distinct advantages as experimental test objects for the following reasons. The first of these is that certain somatic cells of some plant species remain totipotent throughout the life of the plant. This is evidenced by reports that have recently appeared indicating that the progeny of single differentiated somatic plant cells or small groups of such cells may give rise to an entire organism under appropriate environmental conditions (483, 525). A second advantage is the unique manner in which dicotyledonous plant species grow. Primary growth of such plant species results from the rapid division, subsequent elongation, and finally differentiation of the meristematic cells that are found at the extreme apex of a shoot or root. By combining the properties of totipotency and unique growth characteristics it was possible to achieve regularly a recovery of the crown gall tumor cell and thus gain insight into the nature of the heritable cellular change.

The typical crown gall tumor cell possesses a pronounced capacity for proliferation and a very limited capacity for differentiation, but lacks entirely the ability to organize structures such as roots, leaves, or buds. If, however, totipotential cells of certain dicotyledonous plant species are transformed to a moderate degree but not fully, then a morphologically very different type of growth results (77). Such a new growth, or teratoma, contains, in addition to unorganized tumor cells, a chaotic assembly of tissues and organs that show varying degrees of morphological development.

Sterile tissue fragments isolated from abnormal but organized structures found on the teratomas grow profusely and indefinitely, as do typical unorganized crown gall tumor cells, on a basic culture medium that does not support the growth of normal cells of the type from which the tumor cells were derived. Teratoma tissue differs from typical crown gall tumor tissue in that it retains indefinitely in culture a pronounced capacity to organize highly abnormal leaves and buds. Such tumors are transplantable (see Fig. 10). That these teratomas are composed entirely of tumor cells and not of a mixture of normal and tumor cells was demonstrated unequivocally by isolating a number of clones and demonstrating that teratoma tissues of single cell origin behaved in every respect as did the teratoma tissue from which they were derived (81). These clones were isolated from teratoma tissue that had been carried continuously in culture for more than five years.

Since teratoma tissues of single cell origin possessed a capacity to

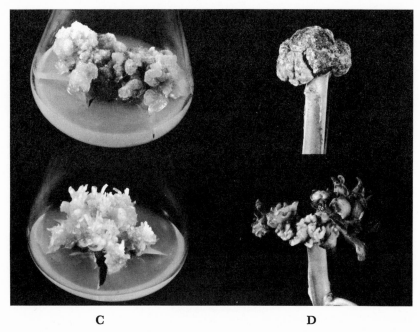

Fig. 10. A. Culture of typical crown gall tumor tissue of tobacco. **B.** Result obtained when a fragment of sterile tumor tissue of the type shown in **A** was grafted to the cut stem end of a tobacco plant. **C.** Culture of crown gall tobacco teratoma tissue of single cell origin. **D.** Result obtained when a fragment of sterile teratoma tissue was grafted to the cut stem end of a tobacco plant.

organize tumor buds, they were admirably suited and were used for studies dealing with the nature of the heritable cellular change that leads to a capacity for autonomous growth of the crown gall tumor cell. In those studies it was hypothesized that if tumor shoots derived from abnormal tumor buds found on the teratomas could be forced into rapid but organized growth, a recovery from the tumorous state might occur regularly if the primary cellular change leading to autonomy was of an epigenetic type but not if it involved somatic mutation at the nuclear gene level since mutations are not believed to be reversed as a result of rapid growth.

In those studies teratoma tissue of single cell origin was grafted onto the cut stem tip of a suitable host plant. The teratoma tissue grew profusely and highly abnormal-appearing leaves and shoots developed. The shoots were removed and were grafted again to the cut stem tip of a healthy host. Such tumor shoots commonly grew very slowly and very abnormally. Tissues isolated from all fleshy parts of such shoots grew well on a simple selective culture medium, indicating that they had retained their tumorous properties. After such shoots reached a height of four to six inches the tips were removed and grafted a second time. Those shoots grew better and were more normal in appearance. When this procedure was followed a third time, it commonly resulted in a completely normal-appearing scion which flowered and set fertile seed. When such seed was sown it gave rise to plants that were normal in every respect. The recovery process is shown in Figure 11. Recovery was thus complete. It was a gradual process that progressed in the direction of the normal as the tumor shoots were forced into rapid but organized growth as the result of a series of tip graftings to healthy plants. Here, then, a reversal of the neoplastic state seems to have been effectively and conclusively demonstrated.

The results of these studies indicate that the crown gall tumor cell contains all of the essential factors both genetic and nongenetic that were present in the normal cell. Nothing had been lost or permanently rearranged as a result of the transformation process. These studies make somatic mutation at the nuclear gene level appear highly unlikely. Since the nuclei in the normal and tumor cells are genetically equivalent—and that is the most important point shown by the recovery studies—the results indicate that we are dealing in this instance with epigenetic modifications which are concerned with a change in the expression of the genetic potentialities that are normally present in a cell. The biosynthetic systems that lead to autonomous growth are gradually and progressively derepressed during the transformation process (see Chapter III), while those systems are again gradually repressed during the recovery phase.

It should be emphasized in passing that the progeny of a single totipotential tumor cell, like an activated egg cell, possesses all of the potentialities required to reconstitute an entire organism with its many different cell types. The inherent potentialities for remodeling metabolic patterns that are present in such cells and the ability of those cells to express those potentialities under appropriate environmental

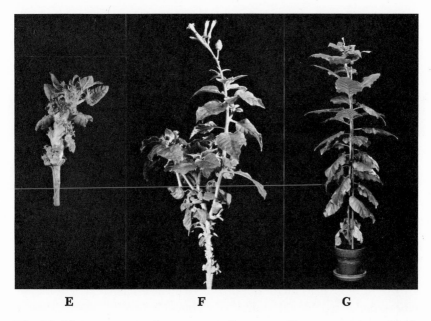

E F G

Fig. 11. Three stages in the recovery of crown gall teratoma tissue. **E.** A tumor bud such as is shown at top right of teratoma pictured in Fig. 10, **D,** was grafted to cut stem tip of a tobacco plant. Note the highly abnormal character of the resulting growth. **F.** A tumor shoot of the type shown at the apex of **E** was grafted to the cut stem end of a healthy tobacco plant. Note that this shoot, although highly abnormal at the base, gradually became more normal and ultimately flowered and set seed. **G.** When the seed was sown it gave rise to plants that were normal in every respect. Since the normal tobacco plant shown in **G** was derived from teratoma tissue of single cell origin, these results demonstrate that the progeny of a single somatic cell of tobacco may possess all of the potentialities necessary to reconstitute an entire tobacco plant. These studies demonstrate unequivocally, moreover, that the nuclei of crown gall tumor cells and those of normal cells are genetically equivalent.

conditions are truly remarkable and this should be kept in mind when considering other examples of this type described below.

Kostoff's Hybrid Tumors

A second neoplastic disease of plants that will be considered very briefly is one in which the genetic constitution of the host and, more particularly, of all the cells of the host plays a primary role. No external agency such as, for example, a virus or a tumorigenic chemical appears to be involved in the inception or development of this disease.

If, for example, two plant species such as *Nicotiana glauca* and *Nicotiana langsdorffii* are crossed and the seed of the hybrid sown, the resulting plants commonly grow normally during the period of their active growth and in the absence of irritation. Once such plants reach maturity and terminal growth ceases, a profusion of tumors invariably develops from all parts of the plant (see Fig. 12). All of the living cells of such plants appear to be potential tumor cells and only irritation such as that accompanying a wound is required to set off the neoplastic process. Such hybrid species appear in reality to be highly organized tumors.

Sterile tumor tissue from such hybrids commonly grows profusely, indefinitely, and in an unorganized manner on a simple culture medium that does not support the growth of cells isolated from either of the non-tumor-producing parents. That the basis for autonomous growth of those cells might not be due to nuclear change of a mutation type is indicated by the studies of White (554). This worker found that when the hybrid tumor tissue was grown on a simple, chemically defined culture medium solidified with agar, it grew indefinitely in a typical unorganized manner. However, when such tissue was immersed in the same culture medium without agar for an extended period of time, the tumor tissue organized normal-appearing shoots and leaves (see Fig. 12). Although these structures were beautifully organized and contained well-differentiated cells, they were not normal since irritation of one sort or another set them off again on a neoplastic course. It is nevertheless possible, in this instance, to switch the pattern from neoplastic to organized growth by simply changing the environment in which the tissues are placed.

Although White (554) initially believed that organization of the tumor tissue resulted from reduced oxygen tension, it can now be surmised from the work of Skoog and his associates (455, 456) that whether such tissue organizes or grows in an unorganized manner is determined in large part by the ratio in the tissues of two plant hormones, the auxins and the cytokinins. High auxin to cytokinin ratios lead to neoplastic growth; the reverse, to organization. This, then, appears to be a problem of development in which the pattern of growth is determined by the ratio of two growth-regulating substances produced in tissues grown under different environmental conditions.

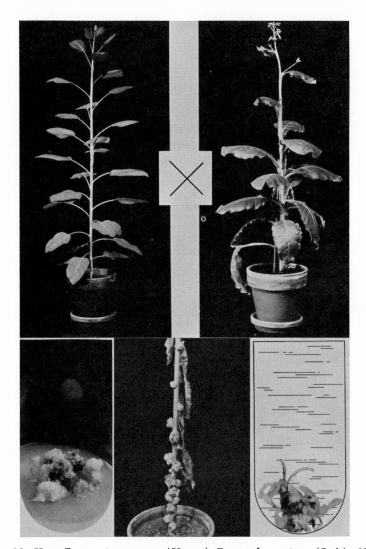

Fig. 12. Kostoff genetic tumors. (*Upper*) Parental species: (*Left*), *Nicotiana glauca*. (*Right*), *Nicotiana langsdorffii*. (*Below, center*), F₁ hybrid. When the hybrid plant reaches maturity a profusion of tumors invariably develops from all parts of the plant. (*Lower left*), Sterile tumor tissue planted on White's basic culture medium solidified with agar grows in a typical unorganized manner. (*Lower right*), When similar tumor tissue is immersed in White's basic medium without agar the tumor tissue organizes leaves and shoots. Thus, the potentialities for organization are retained by the tumor cells.

Reversal of Tumor Growth in Amphibians

In 1935 Waddington (533) and one year later Needham (370) suggested that the autonomy of tumors originates in a "morphological escape" of tumor cells from the controlling influence of an individuation field which has locally become weak or which may be absent. The main characteristic of an individuation field is that all tissues lying within it tend to develop into a complete embryo and in any one part of the field all tissue tends to be built up into the organ corresponding to that part. Needham (371) has suggested that one of the most important aspects of cancerous growth is that it represents an escape from this controlling pattern or field.

In attempting to test this hypothesis it is at once evident that much will depend on the extent to which an individuation field persists in the adult organism. Needham suggests that the power of regeneration may be a suitable measure of this. If that is so, the mammalian individuation field would appear to have been largely lost during development. There are, nevertheless, organisms such as the newt, for example, which possess remarkable powers of regeneration in the adult state. It is well known that in the adult newt the leg area is so potent that it can mold into a limb any mass of competent tissue either grafted into it, or formed on it, as a regeneration bud. Needham has suggested that if suitable amphibian cancerous tissue transplantable onto new tissue could be found, it would be possible to learn whether the autonomously growing cancer cells could be mastered by the individuation field controlling a limb area. It is clear that opportunities for experimental attack along these lines are both numerous and inviting.

Reversal in Frogs

The first published experimental studies designed to test this intriguing idea were carried out by Rose and Wallingford (418). Fragments of the Lucké adenocarcinoma of the leopard frog, *Rana pipiens,* were implanted into regeneration blastemas of limbs of the adult newt *Triturus viridescens.* The results obtained in those studies were interpreted to mean that the Lucké tumor cells had differentiated into muscle, cartilage, and connective-tissue cells. Unfortunately, no unequivocal evidence was presented to indicate that the differentiated cells observed were actually derived from the Lucké tumor. The only criterion used in those studies to distinguish frog and newt cells was the smaller size of the frog nuclei.

Similar and more conclusive experiments of this type were recently carried out by Mizell (362). In order to learn whether tumor cell differentiation was indeed occurring, nuclei of the Lucké tumor were tritium-tagged as a marker. Triteated thymidine was incorporated into the chromosomes of both primary tumors and tumors that were carried as serial intraocular transplants. Fragments of tumors containing tagged nuclei were implanted into the tails of young *Rana pipiens* tadpoles. After the grafts had taken, the tails were amputated through the tumor and the interaction of tumor and host tissue was followed during the regeneration process. Radioautographs of regenerates, which were fixed after various periods of regeneration, revealed the presence of labeled nuclei in several types of normal-appearing cells including muscle, ependymal, fibroblast, and epithelial cells. It thus appears from these studies that the adenocarcinoma cells liberated from the tumor mass following amputation migrate and intermingle with the blastemal cells of the regenerate and, under the influence of the regenerating tissue of the tail, differentiate and mature into cells of various types. If that interpretation of the observations is correct, the results would appear to support the early speculations of Waddington (533) and of Needham (370).

Reversal in Newts

Further studies to test this hypothesis were carried out by Seilern-Aspang and Kratochwil (448, 449) using the European newt *Triturus cristatus* as the experimental test object. The first problem that confronted these workers was to produce experimentally a typical tumor, comparable to malignant tumors in mammals, that could be clearly distinguished from other proliferative processes such as inflammation and regeneration. This they succeeded in doing regularly by injecting carcinogenic hydrocarbons (mixture of 2% dibenzanthracene and 0.2% benzpyrene in olive oil was most effective) subcutaneously. Tumors arose in multicentric fashion from the basal cells of the mucous glands of the skin. These coalesced to form expansively growing tumors which infiltrated and destroyed normal tissues, often penetrating into the peritoneal cavity and metastasizing freely to all parts of the animal. Such tumors were never initiated when irritating but noncarcinogenic substances of various types were similarly applied. In the discussion of their paper the authors raise the question as to whether the new growths are, in fact, comparable to malignant tumors of mammals and conclude from the evidence available that they unquestionably are.

More than half of the animals that developed expansively growing tumors died, indicating the malignant quality of the new growths. In many other instances, however, a most remarkable thing happened. In those instances after the tumors had reached large size, had infiltrated and metastasized, the neoplastic process ended with a spontaneous regression of the tumors. The basis of this regression did not appear to involve death of the tumor cells, but rather a differentiation and maturation of such cells into normal nonmalignant cell types. Within the expansively growing primary tumor neoplastic elements differentiated into pigment cells, typical integumental epithelium, mucous glands, and cornified layers, while the infiltrating portions of the tumor developed into fibrous connective tissue. When cellular differentiation and maturation occurred the animals recovered completely from the disease. Seilern-Aspang and Kratochwil (449) found that they could demonstrate such a recovery most readily by inducing a tumor at a site close to the base of the tail and removing part of the tail to stimulate the regenerative processes in the animals.

Although the inductive factors and other mechanisms by which such morphogenetic transformations occur remain unknown, the results obtained in this system appear to be strikingly similar to those reported for the neuroblastomas of humans which will be considered below. The suggestion seems apparent that the neoplastic transformation in this instance, as in certain of the plant systems, may be a reversible process.

Reversal of the Tumorous State in Mammals

Teratocarcinoma of the Mouse

It might be argued that the newt and the frog, like the plant, are rather low forms of life and that what happens in such lower organisms has really very little to do with what may occur in mammals. What, then, do we know about the occurrence of a spontaneous reversal of the cancerous state in higher forms? A well-documented example of a recovery from the tumorous state is found in the case of a malignant teratocarcinoma of the mouse. This type of tumor typically contains derivatives of all three embryonic germ layers. Such tumors are thought to arise from primitive germ cells or misplaced blastomeres found in or near the ovaries or testes. Those derived from the testes are particularly malignant. Typically, teratocarcinomas, whether found in mice or humans, present a wide variety of cell types. Bone, cartilage, nerve tissue, tooth buds, hair follicles, muscle, as well as other differentiated derivatives may be found to occur in a completely disorganized array. Interspersed among them are groups of essentially undifferentiated cells which are known as embryonal carcinoma cells and which represent the malignant component of the tumor. During serial transfer of such a tumor from mouse to mouse this broad spectrum of cell types is reproduced indefinitely.

Pierce and his associates (393) have carefully analyzed the population dynamics of a complex tumor which arose spontaneously within the testes of a mouse. This tumor, which has been maintained for years by serial transplantation, contains as many as fourteen different, well-differentiated derivatives in addition to embryonal carcinoma cells. It is malignant and when implanted into healthy mice invariably kills the animals in a few weeks' time. In studying the teratocarcinoma, Pierce et al. were interested in learning the origin of the variety of different cell types found in the tumor. Did the various types of cell proliferate independently or did they all arise from a common precursor or stem cell? Initially, Pierce, Dixon, and Verney (393) approached this problem in an indirect and novel way. They injected thick suspensions of the tumor into the peritoneal cavities of mice and obtained many free-floating structures which were called embryoid bodies because of their rather remarkable resemblance to developmental stages of normal ova. The embryoid bodies were initially composed of two or three tissue types, an outer layer of visceral yolk sac, an inner layer of mesenchyme, and, in about one-third of the cases examined, aggregates of embryonal carcinoma cells were imbedded in the mesenchymal tissue.

Pierce et al. (393) studied the developmental potential of neoplastic embryoid bodies by subcutaneous grafting. It was found in those studies that about one-third of the embryoid bodies contained embryonal carcinoma cells at the outset and the same proportion of transplants gave rise to typical teratocarcinomas. The other two-thirds of the implants that lacked embryonal carcinoma cells either disappeared or developed as endodermally lined cysts. Such cysts were found to contain cartilage, muscle, brain, glands, as well as other specialized derivatives. They invariably developed as benign masses. The impression gained from those studies was therefore that embryonal carcinoma cells are not present in such cysts because they have completely differentiated into a variety of specialized and benign cell types.

A crucial experiment designed to examine that problem further was recently reported by Kleinsmith and Pierce (292). These investigators implanted single embryonal carcinoma cells into the peritoneal cavities of mice. It was found that in those approximately fifty instances in which the single cells grew, malignant tumors developed and killed the animals in a few weeks' time. The tumors consisted, however, of the typical mixture of differentiated cell types together with the undifferentiated embryonal carcinoma cells. That is to say, the single cancer cells had given rise not only to embryonal carcinoma cells but to as many as fourteen well-differentiated cell types that were completely benign. These studies clearly demonstrate, then, that a cancer cell in a mammal can give rise to benign or normal derivatives. In other words, the embryonal carcinoma cell is a multipotential cell, highly malignant in the undifferentiated state but capable of giving rise to cells of various types that have lost their malignant properties.

Epidermoid (Squamous) Carcinoma of the Rat

The author had occasion during the early summer of 1968 to visit the laboratory of Professor Roy E. Albert of the Institute of Environmental Medicine of the New York University Medical Center. There he was shown pathological sections and pictures of sections of epidermoid (squamous) carcinomas which had been induced in the skin of rats by ionizing radiation. During discussions of this problem Dr. Albert stated that measurements of the depth of radiation required to induce the formation of these cancers indicated that it was the basal cells of the surface epidermis or of the hair follicles that were trans-formed.

It is, of course, well known that normal basal cells divide giving rise to one derivative that differentiates while the other member of the pair retains the potentialities of the basal cell from which it was derived. Structurally these epidermoid carcinomas consist of an agglomeration of epidermal cell pegs in a matrix of connective tissue (see Fig. 13). Division occurs amongst the tumor cells that form the rim of each peg, while the interior of a peg is composed of cells hav-ing a pattern of differentiation which appears to result from the same keratinizing processes that normally occur in the surface epithelium of the skin. The cells that form the core of the peg show pycnotic nuclei, are heavily keratinized, do not appear to divide, and thus seem to have reached the end of the line as far as further growth and development are concerned.

It is tempting to speculate, therefore, that in this instance the can-cer cell, like the normal basal cell from which it was derived, retains the potentiality to produce differentiated derivatives. This may, there-fore, represent another example to show that those abnormalities which are characteristic of tumor cells do not necessarily include the complete elimination of normal modes of differentiation. The fact that metastases from squamous cell carcinomas may contain, in addition to characteristic tumor cells, differentiated keratinized cell types ap-pears to lend credence to that interpretation. If that interpretation is correct, then it is clear that the potentialities for differentiation reside in cancer cells of this type and the problem resolves itself simply into learning how to bring about the controlled expression of those poten-tialities in all cells of the tumor.

Role of Embryonic Inductors and RNA. One approach to the problem of the controlled differentiation of tumor cells would be the applica-tion of embryonic inductors to such cell types. While such an ap-proach has not as yet received wide attention, certain reports dealing with this matter are found in the literature. For example, de Lustig and Lustig (147) have recently reported the results of studies dealing with the inductive action of chick blastoderm in the primitive streak stage on the differentiation of sarcoma 180 and mouse mammary carcinoma cells. These workers found that under the influence of the

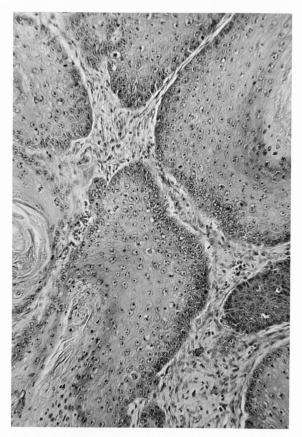

Fig. 13. Section of an epidermoid (squamous) carcinoma of the rat skin induced by ionizing radiation. Structurally, the tumor consists of an agglomeration of branching epidermal cell pegs in a matrix of connective tissue. Division occurs in the tumor cells forming the rim of each peg. The centers of each peg are composed of heavily keratinized cells that no longer appear capable of division. (Courtesy of Dr. Roy E. Albert.)

inductor both types of tumor cells differentiated to form secretory tubules with basement membranes. They also reported that the chorda and neural tube of a 3½-day chick embryo stimulated bone differentiation in a giant cell bone tumor. Of interest was the finding that the inductive effect was still evident when the normal embryonic tissue was separated from the tumor cells by a vitelline membrane. The treated cells retained, in part at least, their tumorous properties in these studies. This could perhaps have resulted from the fact that not all cells of the tumor responded to the inductive stimuli.

It is, nevertheless, clear that the differentiation of tumor cells is not in itself sufficient to insure the loss of tumorous properties. Since a rather elaborate organization of structure and function is quite consistent with the neoplastic state, it is necessary completely and persistently to replace the pattern of synthesis that determines neoplastic growth with that involved in differentiated function if a true reversal of the tumorous state is to be achieved.

A similar although in principle a somewhat different approach to tumor therapy has recently been attempted by Niu (376, 377). This investigator studied the effects of RNA extracted from various sources on the growth of Nelson ascites tumor cells in the mouse. Niu observed that while 96% of control mice injected with the ascites cells developed massive tumors in several weeks' time, preincubation of such cells with calf liver RNA decreased the number of tumors formed to less than 10%. In order to eliminate a possible nonspecific effect of RNA on tumor growth, a control inoculum of ascites cells treated with RNA extracted from the tumor itself was used. In this instance 71% of the animals developed tumors. In the ascites tumor cells treated with calf liver RNA the nodules were found to be smaller than were the controls and the normal anaplastic appearance of the tumor cells was modified by a tendency toward cell groupings and pattern formation.

The striking effects of RNA on tumor growth have now been confirmed in two other laboratories using Novikoff mouse hepatoma (144) and a murine mucous carcinoma of the liver (10). The results obtained with the use of the Novikoff hepatoma were particularly interesting not only because the hepatoma cells treated with liver RNA showed a sixfold decrease in tumor-forming ability but also because the tumors that did develop were far more highly organized than were the untreated control tumors. The cells of the treated tumors tended to organize and radiate around a vein and showed a polarized distribution of glycogen similar to that found in the normal liver. The specificity of the effects of liver RNA was clear since RNA extracted from the tumor or from normal spleen and kidney showed no effects on the growth of the tumor.

Although these are encouraging preliminary results and appear to demonstrate that RNA of foreign origin may penetrate animal cells and serve as messengers to influence the growth and perhaps the developmental potentialities of a cell, a great deal more work will have to be done and much will have to be learned before this type of approach can be applied directly to the tumor problem as a practical therapeutic measure.

Reversal of the Malignant State in Humans

Spontaneous Regressions of Neuroblastomas

The clinical evidence for the spontaneous regression of malignant neoplasms in humans is now considerable. Everson and Cole (174) in their monograph *Spontaneous Regression of Cancer* list 176 well-documented instances of this type. It is clear, moreover, from that report that by no means are all such regressions due to immune or allergic reactions, endocrine influences, unusual sensitivity to usually inadequate therapy, or interference with the nutrition of the cancer. In some instances, as may perhaps best be illustrated by the neuroblastomas of man, regression may involve a maturation and differentiation of cells of both primary and metastatic tumors into highly differentiated ganglion cells that have lost their malignant properties. The incidence of spontaneous regression of such tumors is commonly considered to be very low. However, Koop, Kiesewetter, and Horn (295) in a series of 44 cases found that recovery occurred in 7 cases or 16% of that series. Similarly, Dargeon (140) noted that among 28 patients who survived for 5 years or more, 11 did not receive adequate therapy either by surgery or irradiation. These last two reports suggest that the real incidence of the spontaneous regression of a neuroblastoma may possibly be higher than is commonly believed.

The neuroblastoma is a solid, highly malignant tumor that is apparently derived during organogenesis from the primitive and presumably multipotential sympathetic nerve cell, the neuroblast. Generally the tumor is diagnosed during the first year of life and may even develop prenatally. In the vast majority of patients with untreated neuroblastomas, metastases soon develop and there is a rapid downhill course culminating in death within a few months. There are striking exceptions to this, however. In 1927 Cushing and Wolbach (138), in a carefully studied and now classic case covering many years, reported the conversion of a malignant metastasizing paravertebral sympathicoblastoma into a benign ganglioneuroma composed of apparently mature ganglion cells.

In 1921, ten years after the first exploratory operation and diagnosis had been made, the eminent surgeon Dr. Harvey Cushing performed a laminectomy (138). A sharply demarcated extradural mass of dense noninfiltrating and nonadherent tumor tissue was found which encircled and constricted the meninges and cord. An intraspinal tumor was also exposed. The tumors were removed surgically. Many histological sections were examined and a diagnosis of ganglioneuroma was made by Dr. S. B. Wolbach. Histological sections made in 1911 from the original tumor were also examined by Wolbach at that time and he concurred with the diagnosis of sympathetic neuroblastoma. There may perhaps be some disagreement as to whether this case should be considered an instance of spontaneous regression since the patient was treated with Coley's toxin for a period of time after the initial diagnosis was made. However, authorities today would not consider Coley's toxin to be an acceptable method of therapy.

More recently another case report covering many years and dealing with the conversion of a metastasizing neuroblastoma into a benign ganglioneuroma was recorded in detail by Visfeldt (531). In addition, Everson and Cole (174) list twenty-nine cases of spontaneous regression of neuroblastomas in man. Many other cases of recovery following radiation therapy have been recorded.

Reversal of Neuroblastoma Cells in Culture

It has been found, moreover, that the conversion of neuroblastoma cells into ganglion cells may be accomplished under controlled conditions in culture. Goldstein, Burdman, and Journey (207) cultivated neuroblastoma cells from 13 young children *in vitro* for periods of one week to over a year. All but one of the biopsies contained undifferentiated masses of immature neuroblasts. *In vitro* cultivation of the neuroblastoma cells resulted in differentiation and maturation into more mature neural elements within 5 months. Explantation of the more mature-appearing neuroblastoma cells resulted in the conversion of all of those cells into mature ganglion cells within 20 days.

The increasing number of reports of children who have recovered spontaneously from neuroblastomas as well as the tissue culture studies indicate that the differentiation and maturation of malignant neuroblasts into highly differentiated ganglion cells that have lost their malignant properties can and do occur. We have here, then, a tumor population whose progeny have the potentialities to differentiate and mature.

The Role of the Multipotential Cell
in Understanding the Tumor Problem

It is clear from the selected examples described above that a reversal of the neoplastic state may and does occur in a wide spectrum of organisms ranging from higher plants to newts, frogs, mice, and humans. That phenomenon would appear, therefore, to have broad biological implications. The diverse tumors in which recovery has been demonstrated doubtless have quite different and distinct proximate causes although these are not known in all instances. The common denominator is not, therefore, the proximate cause but rather the multipotential cell that has, in all of these cases, been transformed into a tumor cell.

Why is it, then, that multipotential or other immature cells may recover from the tumorous state while most cancer cells do not? The answer to that question would appear to rest in the fact that multipotential cells are endowed with broad morphogenetic or regenerative capacities. Such cell types can very effectively remodel metabolic patterns as is clearly evident from the results described above. The apparent irreversibility of the tumorous state in the vast majority of instances may simply reflect an inability of most differentiated cell types to undergo intracellular regenerations of the type that are characteristic of a multipotential cell. In other words, the fate of differentiated cells is often strongly determined prior to their transformation and the developmental potentialities of such cells are thus severely restricted. The ultimate fate of the multipotential cells, on the other hand, is essentially undetermined at the time of their transformation and such cell types retain potentialities for development in any one or more of a number of different directions. The cellular mechanism(s) underlying tumorigenesis could very well be and doubtless is the same in the two kinds of cell, and whether or not a recovery from the tumorous state results depends upon the inherent potentialities for remodeling metabolic patterns possessed by each of them.

The several examples of recovery described above will very likely be considered by some to represent special and unique cases and, hence, to be of little relevance to an understanding of the tumor problem generally. It is, nevertheless, true that it is often through an understanding of such special cases that insight is gained into complex biological phenomena. What, then, can be learned from those systems?

It is clear, first of all, from a study of such examples that tumorigenesis need not necessarily involve a change in the integrity of the genetic information that is normally present in a cell. It would be difficult, indeed, to accept the explanation that reversions, which occur regularly in some tumor systems, represent a controlled series of back mutations. Such reversions occur much too frequently to be accounted for by random back mutations which in themselves are relatively rare events. It is apparent from these studies as well as from studies dealing with the hybridization of normal somatic cells and tumor cells described earlier that a deletion of essential genetic information is not etiologically involved in tumorigenesis, at least not in the systems studied. The experimental demonstration of a reversal of the neoplastic state provides, on the other hand, the best evidence yet available to indicate that the cancerous state may be mediated through purely epigenetic mechanisms. Such studies suggest, therefore, that the tumor problem may be basically a problem of anomalous differentiation and that neoplastic growth, like normal developmental processes, stems from epigenetic modifications against a constant cellular genome. This concept might have greater appeal if the normalization of tumor cells could be demonstrated to exist in systems other than those involving multipotential or other immature tumor cell types.

Reversal of Neoplastic Growth in Other Systems

Rous Sarcoma

Examples of a reversal of the tumorous state other than those involving multipotential cells have been recorded in the literature. In a recent study, Macpherson (330) transformed hamster cells of the BHK21 C13 line with the Schmidt-Ruppin strain of the Rous sarcoma virus. The transformed cells, in contrast with uninfected cells of the same type, formed colonies in agar suspension cultures, grew on glass in disarray, and produced tumors in high percentage when implanted into cheek pouches of young adult hamsters.

Five large colonies of transformed cells were selected and single cells were isolated from one of these. Three of 16 single cells isolated formed colonies which were designated as C13/SR1, C13/SR2, and C13/SR3. When grown on glass, all 3 clones formed randomly oriented cell layers indicating that they were composed of transformed cells. C13/SR1 cells grew slowly in culture, while those of the other 2 clones grew rapidly and made the medium very acid. When cells of the 3 clones were plated separately, a small proportion of the C13/SR2 and C13/SR3 cells formed colonies with well-defined parallel orientation similar to those produced by the uninfected cells. Such colonies were considered to be revertants. (See Fig. 14.) Cells of clone C13/SR1 remained 100% transformed but after two passages the cells degenerated and were lost. Clone C13/SR2 attained a stable distribution of colony forms. In seven platings at weekly intervals about 6% of the colonies were found to be revertants. In the case of C13/SR3 the proportion of revertant colonies increased from 5.5% to 19% after 3 weeks and ultimately to 98% after 8 weeks.

Transplantations of the C13/SR clones and subclones were made intradermally into cheek pouches of young adult hamsters. The results of those studies showed that the very low transplantability of the original uninfected C13 cells is very significantly increased by the viral transformation and that the revertant cells had again lost this increased transplantability. The viral content of the transformed and revertant cells was also tested by inoculation into chickens, by serological studies, and by electron microscopy. Although the presence of virus was readily demonstrated in the transformed cells by the three methods, no virus could be demonstrated in any of the revertants. Macpherson concluded from this study that it is possible that reversion in this instance is correlated with the partial or *complete* loss of the RSV genome carried by the transformed cells. If that is so, then the results reported above would suggest that the presence of the RSV genome is essential for the maintenance of the neoplastic state in this system and that a partial or complete loss of that genome results in the recovery of a cell.

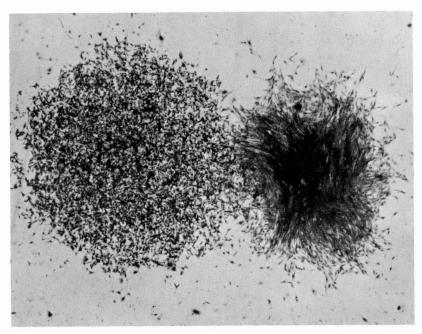

Fig. 14. (*Left*), A colony derived from cloned hamster cells transformed by the Schmidt-Ruppin strain of the Rous sarcoma virus. (*Right*), A revertant colony derived from the cloned transformed cells. The results of these studies suggest that the presence of all or part of the Rous sarcoma virus genome is essential for the maintenance of the neoplastic state. (Courtesy of Dr. Ian Macpherson.)

The Oncogenic DNA Viruses

A situation comparable in certain respects to that reported by Macpherson for Rous-virus-transformed cells may also hold for SV40- and polyoma-transformed mammalian cells. Pollack, Green, and Todaro found that when cloned populations of transformed cells were treated with 5-fluoro-2-deoxyuridine (FUdR) the growing cells were killed but the nonreplicating members of the population were unaffected and thus progeny of the latter could be obtained selectively (399). Among those progeny were found variants that were persistently different from the original population. These progeny possessed both a greatly reduced tumor-forming ability *in vivo* and showed significantly more contact inhibition in culture. Interestingly enough, some viral functions such as the T antigens continued to be present in the "revertant" cells.

Rabinowitz and Sachs (409a), using a different method, have very recently obtained similar results with cells transformed by the polyoma virus. In those studies, clones of cells in which the transformed state had become a hereditary cellular property produced a high frequency of revertants. The reversion in this instance, as in the example cited above, was not associated with the loss of the virus genome. The results of those studies suggest that properties characteristic of transformed cells may or may not be expressed after polyoma virus transformation and that once the expression of those properties has been induced, it can again be repressed. Thus, even with the DNA-containing viruses, the expression of neoplastic behavior is not permanently fixed but is subject to change. The authors of that paper also state that reversion of tumor cells transformed by nonviral carcinogens has been achieved in their laboratory.

Cell Culture Studies

In addition to the numerous reports in the literature concerning the development of tumor cells from normal cells under cultural conditions, there are also reports of tumor cell lines which, when maintained in cell culture for prolonged periods of time, lose the ability to produce tumors when implanted into an appropriate host (184). Essentially two explanations have, in the past, been proposed to deal with such observations. The first of these is that after extended culture antigenic changes occur in the tumor cells, thus leading to an immunological rejection of the cells when implanted into a host. Although changes of this type may indeed occur in certain instances, such an explanation is not in itself always sufficient to account for the loss of tumor-forming ability, since such a loss can also be demonstrated when cultured cells are implanted into newborn, irradiated, or cortisone-treated animals (269). It has therefore been suggested as an alternative explanation that following prolonged culture the tumor cells are overgrown and eventually replaced by normal cell contaminants.

The recent studies of Foley and Drolet (184) would tend to cast doubt on that interpretation since those investigators used a characteristic metabolic marker to follow the identity of the original tumor cells. These workers found that after prolonged culture the sarcoma 180 cells lost their ability to produce tumors when implanted into a suitable host. Such cells still possessed a decreased tryptophan requirement which was the metabolic marker used to distinguish them from normal cells.

It thus appears quite likely that malignant cells have actually reverted in some instances to the nonmalignant state under conditions of cell culture. It would be of interest, therefore, to learn what environmental factors are at work under conditions of cell culture which promote this tendency toward reversion.

Stem Cell Theory

If it is true that certain tumor cells retain the capacity to differentiate into benign cells, it is conceivable that all tumors are actually composed of a heterogeneous population of cells. It is clear that the cell of origin of the tumor would in large part determine the type of differentiation that the tumor cell could undergo. In the teratomas described above, where the cell of origin is a multipotential cell, it is not surprising to find that histological differentiation occurs in many different directions. However, in tumors that arise from differentiated cells, maturation and differentiation might be more difficult to recognize microscopically. These ideas on the heterogeneity of a tumor cell population, which are clearly related to the phenomenon of the differentiation of malignant into benign cells, were proposed a decade or so ago in the form of the stem cell theory by Makino (333, 334, 335). This concept was originally developed to account for the variable karyotypes that are found so commonly in transplantable tumors. It was postulated that certain cells of variant karyotype produced by the stem cells were no longer capable of uncontrolled cell division, and hence were no longer malignant. Thus, the stem cells, like the multipotential tumor stem cells, were postulated to give rise not only to more stem cells but to nonmalignant cells as well.

With the development of techniques for the cloning of cells from a complex tumor population the stem cell theory could be approached experimentally. As a result of their studies on cloned ascites tumors of the mouse, Hauschka and Levan (230) concluded that the stem cell theory required some modification. These investigators found that the tumors studied were frequently composed of multiple cell lines, more than one of which was capable of continuous proliferation. These studies did not, however, shed light on the critical point as far as the present discussion is concerned. They did not answer the question as to whether the stem cells were capable of differentiation into nonmalignant cell types.

The studies of Stich and Steele (486) appear, however, to provide support for that concept. These workers used microspectrophotometric methods to determine the DNA content of individual cells in human neoplasms. The advantage of this method is that while karyotypic analyses are essentially limited to a study of metaphase cells, DNA content can be determined at any point in the cell cycle. When an adenocarcinoma of the stomach was analyzed with the use of this method interesting results were obtained. The DNA content of all metaphase cells was about the same, while an analysis of interphase cells showed a wide scatter of DNA content, much greater than could be accounted for by differences in the doubling time of DNA. Since these widely varying DNA contents were never observed in metaphase cells, the results suggest that within this tumor there exists a population of cells which do not enter mitosis. DNA analyses of other human tumors, although complicated by the presence of multiple cell lines entering mitosis, consistently showed the presence of cell populations which did not divide. The results of these experiments appear to provide further evidence, then, in support of the concept that malignant cells may lose the capacity to divide and hence would no longer be malignant.

The model systems described above provide evidence, then, in support of the belief that the malignant transformation generally may be a potentially reversible event. Despite this evidence, the concept of reversibility of the tumorous state will doubtless meet with strong resistance from many quarters. It may well be argued by some that since the malignant state is by definition an irreversible state, the examples of reversibility cited above cannot possibly be concerned with true tumors because the cells comprising the tumors regularly give rise to benign or normal progeny and, hence, such cells could not be irreversibly altered and are therefore not cancerous. The fallacy of this type of reasoning can perhaps best be illustrated with a story that is attributed to Dr. Peyton Rous. In 1911, after Dr. Rous had reported his findings concerning the viral causation of the fowl sarcoma that bears his name, cancer was by the then accepted definition a disease of unknown etiology. Shortly after Dr. Rous's discovery, an eminent foreign pathologist visited him and, learning firsthand of the studies, turned to Dr. Rous and said: "But, my good man, don't you see it can't be a cancer because you have found the cause."

If cancer cells are, then, not necessarily altered in an irreversible manner and can, in some cases at least, undergo spontaneous differentiation which leads to the production of benign or normal cells, it becomes apparent that learning to control the processes of differentiation in neoplastic cells is important and could, theoretically at least, hold the key to an entirely new approach to cancer therapy. Possible control mechanisms will therefore be considered in the next chapter.

CHAPTER VII

Gene Regulation and Oncogenesis

In view of the results recorded in the previous chapter and elsewhere in this book, it is clear that any future attempt to explain all types of oncogenesis must be flexible enough to accommodate the potential reversibility of the tumorous state and thus to recognize, as has seldom been done in the past, that irreversibility is not the essential feature of that state. The wide spectrum of tumor cell types which have now been demonstrated to be reversible—and which include, among others, cloned teratomas of plant and animal origin, regressions involving the maturation and differentiation of cancer cells in chemically induced tumors in animals and in certain spontaneously arising neuroblastomas in man, the observed loss of the malignant character in tissue culture, the return to normality of cells transformed by the Rous sarcoma virus, the developmental potentialities following the transplantation of tumor nuclei into frog eggs in the case of the Lucké adenocarcinoma, as well as results obtained in studies on the stem cell theory—suggest in the strongest possible manner that the phenomenon of the reversibility of the tumorous state has broad biological implications.

So broad, in fact, is this spectrum of examples that it is tempting to assume that the neoplastic state generally is a potentially reversible process. Implicit in that statement is the concept that stable heritable changes can arise in somatic cells without a change in the integrity of the genetic determinants present in such cells. That such types of heritable changes do, in fact, occur has been thoroughly documented here and elsewhere. The question, then, resolves itself simply into determining which, if any, of one or more of the several different types of heritable cellular change is most likely to be applicable to the tumor problem generally. In order to attempt to answer that question it would seem necessary to analyze the tumor problem in its simplest and most uncomplicated form if the fundamental cellular processes underlying tumorigenesis are to be revealed. This is perhaps best exemplified in the animal field by the type of transplantable tumor described in Chapter I and pictured in Figure 1, which commonly does not invade neighboring tissues and generally does not metastasize but grows to huge size and ultimately causes death by simply overwhelming its host. It is obvious in this instance, as it is so clearly evident in the case of plant tumor systems described here, that a loss of a capacity to regulate the cell division process is fundamental.

The type of tumor pictured in Figure 1 nevertheless occasionally gives rise to derivatives that invade and metastasize. The abilities to invade and to metastasize thus appear to be secondarily acquired characteristics. This is evidenced further by the fact that certain normal cell types such as the macrophages and leukocytes extensively invade tissues and move freely through an organism without producing tumors, because their division mechanism is precisely regulated. This deranged control of cell division in a tumor cell is so widely recognized that many investigators consider it to be the essence of the tumor problem. Nevertheless, Pitot and Cho (395) have recently written:

However, it is apparent that cell division itself is not essential to neoplasia (Fisher and Fisher, 1959) and, probably, that the control of cell division may be essentially normal in a few pathologically defined neoplasms. Two examples of such lesions are the pulmonary hamartoma and the common dermal nevus, both of which grow only as fast as the host tissues (Michael, 1964). Even these few exceptions are most important, for, as has been seen repeatedly in cancer research, any exception to a generalization about neoplasia destroys the generalization.

Pitot and Cho go on to state:

Thus, cell division and probably even the control of cell division are not essential to the nature of cancer, but rather may be manifestations of a more basic molecular change in control mechanisms.

The statements quoted above require careful analysis and critical comment. It is, first of all, not apparent, as Pitot and Cho state, "that cell division itself is not essential to neoplasia." Without cell division there obviously would be no tumors. One would hardly consider a transformed but nonreplicating cell to constitute a tumor. Until such a cell divided and its progeny formed at least a microscopically visible new growth, a tumor would not be considered to exist. A distinction must, therefore, be made between a tumor cell and a tumor which by every accepted definition is "a mass of noninflammatory and independent tissue" (542). Pitot and Cho state further "that the control of cell division may be essentially normal in a few pathologically defined neoplasms." As examples of this they cite the pulmonary hamartoma and the common dermal nevus. These examples do not appear to be sufficiently compelling to discard out of hand the generalization that a deranged control of cell division is the essence of the tumor problem. This is particularly true when it is considered that autonomy is not a fixed and unvarying character but has many gradations ranging from the most rapidly growing to the most slowly growing tumor cell types. It should not be surprising, therefore, to find in this spectrum extreme examples in which control of cell division does not deviate significantly from the normal.

Pitot and Cho state further that the pulmonary hamartoma and the dermal nevus "grow only as fast as the host tissues." As was pointed out in the first chapter of this book, it is not the rate of growth but rather the acquisition of a capacity for autonomous growth that is important to the tumor problem. It was indicated, further, that certain normal cell types such as regenerating liver cells may grow at a faster rate than do hepatoma cells. One might reasonably expect, therefore, that in certain instances the rate of growth of tumor cells and normal cells might be the same. However, because of a capacity for autonomous growth of the tumor cell, the end result would be quite different. There would result in the case of the tumor cells an essentially unorganized mass, and in the normal, beautifully organized cell structures.

It should be pointed out, moreover, that there is not complete agreement among pathologists as to whether the hamartoma should, in fact, be considered a true neoplasm or whether it is merely a malformation that results from defective development of neighboring tissues. At any rate, the hamartoma appears to represent a borderline case. The dermal nevus, like the hamartoma, is a benign growth the size of which commonly does not change significantly over a period of many years. Yet the mere fact that the dermal nevus is recognizable as an abnormal growth indicates a relaxation, however slight and however temporary that may be, of control over the growth of its cells.

To argue on the basis of the two examples cited above that "any exception to a generalization about neoplasia destroys the generalization" would appear like insisting that since there are a few unquestioned examples of terminal differentiation, e.g., the mature red blood cell of man which has lost its nucleus, all cellular differentiation must be irreversible. We have seen that that is not true. Thus there appear at present to be neither good nor valid reasons for not believing that the fundamental biochemical lesion in a tumor cell is one that affects processes concerned with the regulation of cell growth and division.

These fundamental growth processes are controlled, as we have seen, in higher plant species by the quantitative interaction of two growth-regulating hormones, the auxins and the cytokinins. Mitogenic hormones are similarly operative in target cells of animals. In epidermal cells of mammals, on the other hand, and perhaps in certain other cell types as well, regulation appears to be accomplished through a repressor system involving an epidermal chalone and adrenalin. Addition of the hormones in the one case or removal of the chalone-adrenalin complex in the other results in the development of a new pattern of synthesis in a cell, going from the precisely regulated pattern of metabolism concerned with differentiated function, which is characteristic of a normal resting cell, to one involving the production of the nucleic acids and the specialized mitotic and enzymatic proteins, as well as other substances required specifically for cell growth and division.

We can maintain with confidence that the key mechanisms involved in the production of these new and specialized products required for cell division act through the processes and components of the gene action system which is ubiquitous in its fundamental aspects and is thus common to cell types generally. Information on the components of the gene action system presented below was obtained in part from a discussion of that subject by K. C. Atwood in *Reproduction: Molecular, Subcellular, and Cellular* (M. Locke, ed.), p. 17, Academic Press, New York and London, 1965.

The Gene Action System

The underlying basis of the organization of the gene action system is that, except for the RNA viruses, the only part of the system that specifies itself is DNA. It logically follows, therefore, that all other macromolecular species found in a cell are specified by the DNA. Since DNA cannot replicate itself but requires an enzyme or enzyme complex for duplication, it follows further that the synthesis of such an enzyme(s) requires the processes of transcription and translation. Transcription, in turn, requires a transcribing enzyme, RNA polymerase, which polymerizes ribonucleoside 5'-triphosphates in the presence of an appropriate template, which is normally double-stranded DNA, of which only one strand is copied, to synthesize the messenger or mRNA which can be translated into protein.

The normal transcription process exhibits two important features, strand selection and chain delineation, the molecular basis of which may ultimately reside in the local sequence characteristics of the DNA being copied. The mRNA, which has a base composition similar to that found in the DNA being copied, is normally translated into protein and may vary in size in a given organism between 8S and 45S. The larger messages are probably polycistronic, i.e., composite transcripts of several genes involved in the synthesis of polypeptide chains. Typically, mRNA is not conserved and in *E. coli*, for example, it persists for approximately 3 minutes, which is time enough to be translated about ten times. In the alga *Acetabularia*, on the other hand, certain mRNA's appear to be highly stable and may persist for many months. Similarly, the hemoglobin mRNA in reticulocytes is relatively stable. The intrinsic characteristics or circumstances that distinguish stable from unstable mRNA remain essentially unknown.

In addition to mRNA two other basic types of RNA are transcribed. The transfer or tRNA's constitute the genetic dictionary and are involved in the selective transport of amino acids to the site of polypeptide synthesis. These RNA's are relatively small and have a molecular weight of about 25,000 and a sedimentation constant of 4S. The minimum number of different kinds of these RNA's present in a cell would be 20, a number corresponding to each essential amino acid, while the maximum number that could be present is 64, the number of codons that can be formed from the four bases. The actual number would be determined by the degree of degeneracy of the genetic code and, from what is now known, the number probably lies near the upper limit.

The tRNA's have two specific recognition sites: the anticodon, which matches complementary trinucleotide codons of the RNA message, and a site recognized by a transfer enzyme that is, in turn, specific for the amino acid signified by the codon. Since the transfer enzymes, like the tRNA's, show specificity it follows that the number of different transfer enzymes in a cell lies somewhere between 20 and 64. However, the number of such enzymes need not necessarily be determined by the number of synonyms for the amino acids. If, for example, the tRNA molecules with synonymous anticodons have the same enzyme recognition site, then the number of transfer enzymes present in a cell could be as few as 20 even if the number of different tRNA's would be as many as 64.

It might be of interest to note here very briefly that certain highly active purine type cytokinins (6-($\gamma\gamma$-dimethylallylamino)purine) of plants have been found to be present in at least two tRNA's, serine and tyrosine, and to be absent in five others studied. Of particular interest was the finding that the cytokinin molecule was immediately adjacent to the anticodon in both the serine and tyrosine tRNA's. This would suggest that its purpose may be to maintain the proper spatial arrangement for the anticodon. Whether the presence of a cytokinin in tRNA has any relation to its biological activity is not known for certain at present, although very recent studies (277) suggest that it may not have. This subject has recently been reviewed in detail by Helgeson (235).

The third class of RNA's formed in a cell are the ribosomal or rRNA's. Typically, two distinct rRNA molecules are distinguishable by their sedimentation constants. In a number of metazoan cells 18S and 28S fragments are found, while in *E. coli* they are characteristically 16S and 23S. In addition to the rRNA's about 35% protein is found in a functional ribosome. The functional ribosome has been compared to a mechanical tape-reading device that moves from one end of the genetic message to the other.

The translation of the genetic message may be subdivided into two stages. The first stage consists of the formation of aminoacyl-tRNA in two steps, which have been termed activation and transfer. Both of these steps are carried out by the same enzyme, the transfer enzyme, which is at one and the same time specific for the amino acid and for an acceptor RNA that has the appropriate codon recognition specificity for its function in stage two.

The second stage of translation, on the other hand, deals with those events that are concerned with the attachment of the tRNA-amino acid complex to a message-ribosome combination. Wettstein and Noll (553) have suggested that there are three ribosomal attachment sites. The first of these is an entrance site to which the charged tRNA is initially attached; the second, a chain-attached site to which the charged tRNA is moved concomitantly with the formation of the peptide linkage between the amino group of its amino acid and the carboxyl end of the polypeptide that is being synthesized; and the third, an exit site which is temporarily occupied by the displaced uncharged tRNA. While the uncharged tRNA is loosely bound to the exit site and is in equilibrium with the uncharged tRNA in solution, both the charged and chain-attached tRNA are tightly bound to their sites if the ionic environment is suitable. The stable binding of charged tRNA to the mRNA-ribosome complex has been found to be dependent on the presence of NH_4^+ or K^+ ions.

Guanosine triphosphate (GTP) and several protein factors extracted from ribosomes (F1 and F2) and from the soluble fraction of the cell (T and G) participate in ribosome-dependent polypeptide synthesis. During this process the GTP is hydrolyzed to GDP and inorganic phosphate. The GTP appears to be involved in a number of steps in the overall reaction. It acts in chain initiation along with the factors F1 and F2 to bind the initiator, N-formylmethionyl tRNA, to the ribosome-mRNA complex. GTP also interacts with the T factor and aminoacyl-tRNA to form a complex that causes the attachment of the aminoacyl-tRNA to the ribosome-carrying mRNA and the chain initiator. GTP hydrolysis is not required for either of these binding reactions. GTP must, moreover, be used in both binding reactions for peptide bond formation to occur between the initiator and aminoacyl-tRNA. Under these conditions GTP hydrolysis is observed. This hydrolysis apparently accompanies some as yet uncharacterized reaction that takes place after the binding steps but before peptide bond formation. GTP and the G factor are involved in the movement of the peptidyl-tRNA and the mRNA on the ribosome. GTP hydrolysis is also observed in this step.

In addition to mRNA, functional ribosomes, and charged tRNA, the second stage of translation requires Mg^{++} and several supernatant protein fractions. It has been suggested that one of these is a peptide polymerase.

Finally, the correct specification of the amino acid at each position in the polypeptide chain depends on the accurate maintenance of the reading frame since, as Crick et al. (134) have pointed out, the code is nonoverlapping. This clearly means that the point of initiation in the second stage of translation is critical in establishing the reading frame for the entire message. Signals for polypeptide chain termination must also be present at appropriate points as part of the message itself. If, as is now generally accepted, DNA is the template which is transcribed in the form of messenger RNA and the messenger associates with ribosomes and it is on the ribosomes that the peptide sequence of a protein is synthesized, then it remains to be stated that the primary one-dimensional structure of the polypeptide that is synthesized determines the secondary and tertiary structure of a protein as a result of the spontaneous folding of the linear peptide. There is, however, still another level of structure of proteins that is important biologically and this is referred to as the quaternary structure. The larger proteins are formed through the spontaneous aggregation of several polypeptides through noncovalent bonding. The biological activity of many proteins is related to this quaternary structure. These important findings suggest, then, that all biological information is carried in a one-dimensional code.

The Regulation of the Gene Action System

The question that arises next is, therefore, How is this gene action system regulated to permit synthesis by a cell of the specialized products required specifically for cell growth and division? The basic cellular mechanisms here appear to be similar to those involved in cellular differentiation in that both instances depend for their expression on the regulation of genes. How, then, are these genes selectively activated and repressed?

It is obvious from what has been reported here that regulatory mechanisms are not one-way avenues of communication out of the nucleus with the rest of the cell playing an essentially passive role. It is clear, furthermore, that it is no longer possible to regard the chromosomes or chromosomal activity as being immune from the environment since the nucleus has been found to be highly responsive to the external conditions in which it operates. The interphase nucleus is, as we have seen, responsive to certain hormonal stimuli, to stress, to changes in nutrition, to ion fluxes, and to inductive effects from neighboring tissues, as well as to certain as yet uncharacterized cytoplasmic factors which have been found to play a central role in the regulation of both the cell division process and cell differentiation. Thus, we see that superimposed on the gene action system are mechanisms whereby transcription or translation of a gene is made conditional on specific stimuli (13). This was first clearly demonstrated by Monod and his associates in their studies on enzyme induction in the bacteria. From those and other studies has emerged the now classic Jacob-Monod scheme (261), which has served as a most useful model for gene regulation in the bacteria. The evidence in support of that scheme derives in large part from genetic evidence related to systems in which exogenous inducing substances control the synthesis of specific enzymes.

This model, described in its briefest form, indicates that the familiar structural genes, that is, those genes that serve as templates for the synthesis of mRNA and ultimately proteins, may be assembled in units of one or more genes which have been named operons. The operon, as a group of functionally related genes, is under the control of a given operator locus, which is sometimes but not always intimately associated with the operon that it controls. The operator locus is, in turn, controlled by a repressor, which is the product of a regulator gene. It is the primary function of a repressor substance to block, through its action on an operator locus, a structural gene(s) that is being regulated or the products of the biosynthetic systems that are being regulated. A repressor molecule, the lactose repressor, which is a product of a regulator gene (*i* gene) in *E. coli,* has now been isolated and found to be a protein having a molecular weight of 150,000 to 200,000; it occurs in a cell at a level of about ten copies per gene (203). Evidence for the existence of regulator genes derives from the mapping of mutations that disturb the response of a cell to an inducer. Such mappings have revealed the presence of regulatory genes at sites distinct from the location of the structural genes.

In addition, another component of a functional operon, the promoter, has been recognized. In the lactose operon of *E. coli,* for example, it has been found that the operator locus is situated outside the first known structural gene from which it is separated by a region that has been called the promoter. The promoter, which probably corresponds to one of the punctuation marks, is indispensable for the expression of the entire operon.

The occurrence of polycistronic operons implies the existence of a double system of punctuation in the nucleic acid text. The first type of punctuation must delimit the long DNA duplex into sections of transcription which correspond to the operons. These punctuation marks thus serve as recognition sites to indicate to the RNA polymerase not only where to start and stop the transcription process but also which of the two strands of the DNA is to be copied. The second type of punctuation in the nucleic acid text is concerned with the division, as it were, of the mRNA in such a way as to correspond to the respective genes in an operon. This type of punctuation serves as a signal to the translating system for delimiting the amino terminal and carboxy terminal ends of the polypeptide chain that is being synthesized.

The really essential point, however, for purposes of this discussion is that this system as visualized operates directly at the genetic level and that in most instances it operates negatively in the sense that when the system of control is active, the corresponding operon is inactive. Thus, inactivation of a repressor activates the operon while activation of the repressor results in the inactivation of the operon. This general scheme of the regulation of gene activity in bacteria by means of repressions and derepressions appears to be firmly based and thus provides a model for that aspect of cell division and cell differentiation that is concerned with the synthesis of new and specialized gene products by different kinds of cells.

It should be pointed out, however, that two objections may immediately be raised. The first of these is that we do not know at this time whether the same types of control mechanisms found in the bacteria are operating in mammalian cells. A second objection that may be raised is that while bacterial regulatory systems of the type described above are entirely reversible, cellular differentiation is by definition a stable phenomenon and instances of terminal differentiation are clearly irreversible. Jacob and Monod (262) recognized this problem and devised a number of rather ingenious circuits based on positive feedback loops that would in principle confer stability on their system. These hypothetical circuits are of importance not only because they provide a model to explain differentiation but also because they show that, in principle at least, it is easy to account for the stabilization of the properties of a given cell type in the presence of a constant cellular genome. These investigators recognized the possible significance of their model systems to cancer when they stated:

These observations may have some bearings on the problem of the initial event leading to malignancy. Malignant cells have lost sensitivity to the conditions which control multiplication in normal tissues. . . . But while the initial event . . . may of course be a genetic mutation, it might also be brought by the transient action of an agent capable of complexing or inactivating *temporarily* a genetic locus, or a repressor, involved in the control of multiplication. It is clear that a wide variety of agents, from viruses to carcinogenes [*sic*], might be responsible for such an initial event (363).

These ideas were further developed by Pitot and Heidelberger (396) who proposed several regulatory models which could specifically explain the induction of a stable malignant state without requiring a permanent alteration in the genetic material present in a cell. In the simplest system the carcinogenic agent can be pictured as temporarily inactivating a specific repressor molecule. Inactivation of this repressor allows the operon which it normally inhibits to become active, and this newly activated operon can, in turn, indirectly inhibit production of the original repressor. Once this stable shift in gene activity occurs, the presence of the carcinogenic agent is no longer necessary to maintain the new steady state. Although the switch in gene activity is stable and can be perpetuated by cell division, it is theoretically reversible. Any agent capable of temporarily repressing the newly activated operon would allow the original steady state to be resumed again. These speculations by Pitot and Heidelberger led them to the conclusion that "if malignancy is not the result of a direct gene (DNA) mutation, a reversion from the malignant to the non-malignant state is well within reason."

Biochemical Aspects of Nuclear DNA Function

This, then, brings us to the question of how the genes in a cell are selectively activated and repressed at the biochemical level in cells of higher organisms. It is, unfortunately, in this most important area that present knowledge is inadequate. While it is true that cellular control processes are varied and may exert their effects at many different levels in a cell, attention here will be focused on the biochemical aspects of nuclear DNA function and its regulation.

The Histones

In considering problems of regulation at the chromosome level it should be recalled that the DNA is present in a chromosome both in an active or diffuse state and in an inactive or condensed form. This suggests that the physical state of the chromatin may somehow be determined by other chromosomal constituents and, more particularly, by the proteins. Of these, a class of basic proteins known as the histones has been intensively studied in that regard. Although for many years the histones were thought to lack specificity and hence were largely ruled out as regulators of gene activity, recent studies have shown that histone fractions differing in chemical composition, including the ratio of arginine to lysine as well as the degree of acetylation, may be obtained from nuclei of different tissues. Such indications of structural specificity are encouraging, and correlation with functional specificity will be described below.

Interest in this area began with the suggestion by Stedman and Stedman in 1951 that histones may act to control gene action (476a). Ten years later Allfrey (11) observed that when histones isolated from thymus nuclei were added to isolated nuclei they inhibited RNA and protein synthesis. This effect was subsequently studied in some detail in the belief that it might lead to a better understanding of the chemical factors controlling chromosomal activity. Among the biochemical activities shown to be inhibited by histones are nuclear ATP synthesis and amino acid transport, as well as amino acid uptake by nuclei and by ribosomes. It should be pointed out, however, that histones are toxic to other enzyme systems such as cytochrome oxidase and they are known to block mitochondrial respiration and phosphorylation. Thus, extreme caution must be exercised regarding the interpretation of specificity of the inhibition of histones on nuclear RNA synthesis.

Huang and Bonner (250) approached the problem of histone function in another way. These workers examined the RNA polymerase activity of DNA fractions isolated from pea-seedling nuclei and observed that free DNA was more effective as a primer or template for RNA synthesis than was DNA containing histones. Similar observations have been made by others (15, 30, 63, 240, 255). Here, too, caution must be exercised in interpreting the findings because similar results may be obtained with other basic proteins and even with certain synthetic polycations. Sonnenberg and Zubay (468), on the basis of their studies, have, in fact, questioned the specific repressor function of the histones.

Still other approaches to this problem have been attempted. Allfrey, Mirsky, and Osawa (17) have found that selective tryptic digestion preferentially removes histones from calf thymus nuclei. Following such treatment, the rate of RNA synthesis may be 300% to 400% higher than that found in the untrypsinized control nuclei. Moreover, the addition of fresh histone to the treated nuclei results in an immediate inhibition of further RNA synthesis. Similarly, Robert and Kroeger (417) have found that trypsin treatment of the polytene chromosomes of insects leads to a significant increase in RNA synthesis in "puff" regions that were already synthesizing RNA. These findings are of interest because (1) they suggest that the active RNA synthesizing loci of chromosomes contain histones, which would argue against the simplistic supposition that DNA function requires complete histone removal, and (2) an increased susceptibility of the histones at RNA synthesizing loci to attack by trypsin indicates that they are less protected than are the histones in the condensed regions of a chromosome. If that is true it raises the distinct possibility that DNA-histone linkages are not fixed but can be modified during the transition from the condensed to the diffuse or active form of DNA.

It is well known, in thymus nuclei at least, that the histones contain acetyl and methyl groups in addition to their amino acid constituents. It has been found, moreover, that both acetylation and methylation of the histones occur after the polypeptide chain has been synthesized. In acetylation the donor group is acetyl coenzyme A, while in methylation it is S-adenosylmethionine. Both are enzymatically controlled processes.

Because of these rather remarkable structural modifications of the histones, comparative studies of the degree of acetylation of different types of histones in resting and activated nuclei were undertaken by Allfrey, Faulkner, and Mirsky (14). When the nuclei were labeled with acetyl coenzyme A-^{14}C it was found that the greatest amount of the label was present in the arginine-rich histone fraction. This fraction had been shown (15) to be a strong inhibitor of the RNA polymerase reaction. These results suggested, then, that because of the high rate of incorporation of acetate into the arginine-rich histones, acetylation might affect the interaction of these proteins with the DNA template.

To test this possibility the histones were isolated, acetylated chemically *in vitro*, and tested in three different RNA polymerase systems. All three systems were found to be somewhat inhibited by the arginine-rich histone fractions but in all instances the artificially acetylated histones failed to inhibit as effectively as did the original histone fraction. This was true despite the fact that the acetylated derivatives were still highly basic proteins with a strong affinity for DNA. They were, moreover, readily taken up by nuclei from which the native histones had been removed. It was concluded from those studies that relatively minor changes in histone chemistry can influence DNA-histone interactions and thus modify the template activity of DNA in an RNA polymerase assay system. This was evidenced by subsequent experiments which demonstrated that histone acetylation, like RNA synthesis, was significantly more pronounced in the diffuse or "active" chromatin fraction than in the condensed or "inactive" fraction (12, 14).

Additional and more direct evidence relating the acetylation of histones to the activity of chromatin was obtained with the use of human peripheral lymphocytes stimulated to divide with phytohemagglutinin, a protein fraction derived from the common garden bean. Human lymphocytes rarely divide in culture, but when such cells are treated with phytohemagglutinin almost all of the cells divide within a 48- to 72-hour period. Isolated lymphocytes maintained in culture for 20 to 24 hours respond almost immediately to the triggering action of the bean protein with the synthesis of new types of RNA and protein. Changes in amino acid incorporation into protein become evident within 15 minutes. Amino acid uptake can be blocked by both puromycin and actinomycin D (397), suggesting that the synthesis of new types of RNA is a prerequisite for the synthesis of new protein.

With the use of this system it was possible to study the metabolism of histones in resting cells and in cells that were preparing to divide. The results of those studies demonstrated that histone acetylation, like RNA synthesis, increases soon after the addition of phytohemagglutinin to the lymphocytes (397). As in the case of the thymus nuclei, the arginine-rich histone fraction showed a greater rate of acetate ^{14}C uptake than did the lysine-rich fraction. It was found, moreover, that the protein-treated lymphocytes acetylate their histones much more rapidly than do the resting control cells. Acetylation of the arginine-rich histone fraction in the treated cells exceeded that of the control cells by as much as 400%.

Even more striking was a comparison of the manner in which acetate uptake into histones and uridine uptake into RNA changed with time following the addition of phytohemagglutinin to the lymphocytes. While the results of such experiments showed that control lymphocytes incorporated acetate into histones or uridine into RNA at an essentially uniform rate over the time period studied, the rate of acetylation in the treated cells increased rapidly with time. The increased rate of histone acetylation appeared, moreover, to precede the increased uptake of RNA precursors. These results were interpreted to mean that a change in the structure of the chromatin brought about by or coincident with histone acetylation is a necessary prerequisite for the synthesis of new RNA's at a previously repressed gene locus.

The Phosphoproteins

Histone acetylation is, of course, only one aspect of the as yet little understood chemistry of chromatin. Other facets of this complex problem that have recently attracted interest are histone methylation and histone phosphorylation, as well as the chromatin-associated phosphoproteins. The phosphoproteins found in the nucleus are of particular interest because, as Allfrey (13) has pointed out, the regions of high negative charge density found in such proteins could influence

DNA-histone interactions and thus modify the structure and function of the chromatin. Indeed, complexes between isolated phosphoproteins and histones can be formed *in vitro* and their formation does reduce the inhibitory effects of added histones on the RNA polymerase reaction (299).

Since RNA synthesis appears to require the template DNA to exist in a diffuse state, one might predict an increase in nuclear phosphorylation during periods of gene activation if the phosphoproteins played a regulatory role. This problem has, in fact, been studied with the use of human lymphocytes triggered to divide with phytohemagglutinin (291). It was found in those studies that the specific activity of the phosphoproteins in the phytohemagglutinin-treated cells was 200% greater than that found in corresponding controls. The kinetics of ^{32}P uptake suggested, moreover, that protein phosphorylation, like histone acetylation, is an early event in the course of gene activation in this system. While suggestive, these results are not yet conclusive since they may have meanings very different from those implied above. Yet, the correlation with gene activation, and the kinetic studies on protein phosphorylation and turnover under varying physiological conditions, appear at this time to be promising leads in this very difficult field of study.

There now appears to be good evidence that there is a change in the soluble nuclear proteins following transformation to the tumorous state. Bakay and Sorof (26) made a detailed electrophoretic study of the soluble nuclear proteins of normal liver and azo-dye-induced hepatomas and found that the tumor cells have less of the basic and near-basic proteins and more of the acidic proteins than do normal liver cells. These interesting results indicate that nuclear charge distributions are altered in the tumor cells and, since charge is one of the major variables affecting DNA-histone interactions, the shift toward negativity could have an influence on the template activity of the DNA. However, it remains to be determined whether such changes in nuclear protein composition are causally involved in genetic control or whether they are merely the result of an abnormal protein metabolism.

Nevertheless, the most fundamental and pressing problem in this area, i.e., an understanding of how RNA synthesis is specifically induced or repressed at a relatively few loci in the chromosomes, does not appear to be readily answerable in terms of histone-DNA interactions. While it is now perfectly clear that different histones can influence the structure of chromatin differently and that histone structure may become modified in the course of gene activation, the problem of the placement of the histones on different cistrons along the DNA double helix remains completely unresolved (13).

According to Allfrey (13), what appears to be required is a control mechanism that permits gene recognition by complementary base pairing between DNA nucleotides and a complementary nucleotide sequence. Such a control mechanism would offer an attractive alternative to the view that proteins alone recognize and influence the function of the many genetic loci in a chromosome, since such a hypothetical control mechanism would involve the delivery and binding of regulatory proteins at sites dictated by the recognition sequences of attached polynucleotides. It may be noted in this connection that there are many reports in the literature of the presence of low molecular weight RNA's in cells of higher organisms and some of these appear to be associated with the proteins of the chromatin (251). Whether such RNA's are significant components of nuclear control mechanisms remains to be determined, however.

The Relevance of Regulatory Mechanisms to the Tumor Problem

How, then, are the regulatory mechanisms that permit the selective activation of the genome of a cell and that permit cells to synthesize new species of RNA relevant to the tumor problem? It has been emphasized throughout this discussion that the transition from a normal resting cell to a persistently dividing tumor cell involves a profound reorientation in the pattern of synthesis in a cell, going from the precisely regulated metabolism concerned with differentiated function, which is characteristic of a normal resting cell, to one involving the synthesis of the specialized products required specifically for continued cell growth and division. This radical and persistent reorientation in metabolism appears, as was pointed out earlier, to be in every way comparable to the persistent switches in metabolism that characterize cellular differentiation during the course of development. In both instances new and specialized products, which commonly have specialized functions to perform, are synthesized by the cells.

The main product found in a persistently dividing cell is, of course, the protein of the mitotic apparatus which is highly specialized in function and may constitute more than 30% of the total protein in certain tumor cell types. It is obvious, therefore, that a persistently dividing cell is "reading" parts of the genome that are ordinarily repressed in a normal resting cell as far as their template activity is concerned. Since these are new and specialized products required specifically for cell growth and division that are being synthesized by persistently dividing cells, it follows that new patterns of RNA synthesis required for the production of the new products must be established and maintained in such cells. Experimental evidence in support of this view comes from the studies of Kidson and Kirby (282) who have shown, by means of countercurrent distribution analysis of rapidly labeled RNA's of normal and hepatoma tissues, that the hepatoma tissue was significantly different from the normal in its spectrum of messenger RNA's. It should be pointed out here, however, that very recently questions have been raised concerning the type of RNA that was actually being measured by Kidson and Kirby. Nevertheless, these investigators (283) reported that the shift away from the normal pattern of RNA synthesis is gradual and becomes more pronounced during prolonged feeding of certain carcinogenic azo dyes. Of great interest was the observation that changes in liver RNA metabolism are reversible if azo-dye feeding is stopped in time. The implication of that finding is, of course, that feedback to the chromosomes may be effective as a control mechanism, at least in an early precancerous state (13).

An attempt has been made here to document, insofar as that is now possible, the premise that the basic cellular mechanisms underlying tumorigenesis are similar in every respect to those underlying the normal processes of cell division and cell differentiation. This concept is particularly well illustrated in the plant tumor systems where the cellular factors involved in the development of a capacity for autonomous growth are far better understood than they are in the animal field. The three plant tumor systems described here have three different and quite distinct proximate causes, an RNA-containing virus in the case of Black's wound tumor disease, a tumor-inducing principle associated with a specific bacterium in the case of the crown gall disease, while simple irritation is all that is needed to initiate neoplasms in the Kostoff hybrid tumors. Yet the end result in all three is the same. In all instances the tumor cells have acquired as a result of their transformation a capacity to synthesize persistently all the metabolites that their normal counterparts require but cannot make for cell growth and division. The continued production of these key metabolites by plant tumor cells keeps those cells dividing persistently.

Thus, three different and quite distinct proximate causes can bring about essentially the same end result. The evidence indicates, moreover, that all three of the proximate causes act in a cell by bringing about, perhaps in different ways, a persistent activation of biosynthetic systems that are concerned with cell growth and division. The fact that a controlled recovery from the neoplastic state has been achieved experimentally in two of the three instances indicates that the nuclei of the normal and tumor cell types are genetically equivalent, thus demonstrating that deletion or permanent rearrangement of the genetic information present in a cell is not an essential prerequisite for the establishment of the tumorous state.

It is interesting to note, moreover, that in the case of the hybrid plants that give rise to the Kostoff genetic tumors the regulatory mechanisms controlling growth and development are so unstable that simple irritation is all that is required to establish and maintain persistently the pattern of metabolism in a cell that is characteristic of the neoplastic state. Thus, in this instance at least, one does not have to postulate the addition, deletion, or permanent rearrangement of genetic information in a cell to account for the tumorous state. One does not even need to postulate the presence in cells of special cancer genes, as has sometimes been done, for it has been shown that all that is required is the persistent activation of biosynthetic systems that are normally concerned with cell growth and division. In those cell types in which the regulatory mechanisms are more stable than in the *Nicotiana* hybrids, exogenous agencies appear to be needed to bring about a persistent activation of those biosynthetic systems. The fact, moreover, that the same two substances that normally regulate cell growth and division (see Fig. 3) are etiologically involved in establishing the tumorous state in plant cells (see Fig. 4) and are also importantly concerned in morphogenesis (see Fig. 8) indicates in the strongest possible manner that the tumor problem, in plants at least, is simply an extreme aspect of the larger problem of development.

If, as now seems likely, that is true of tumors generally, then it would appear necessary to be able to manipulate nuclear function at will if that concept is to be exploited therapeutically. While such a goal may at first sight seem most remote, there is every reason to believe that in the not too distant future new approaches and techniques will be developed and thus become available for selectively influencing nuclear activity. There is certainly no longer any valid reason for believing that chromosomal activity is beyond hope of correction (13). Moreover, there now seems little question that that is precisely what is happening under natural conditions in multipotential tumor cells of both plant and animal origin during the reversal of the neoplastic state. The most striking examples of the possibilities offered by such an approach are, of course, the well-documented cases of the neuroblastomas of man in which the highly malignant and metastasizing neuroblastoma cells matured and differentiated spontaneously into ganglion cells that had lost their malignant properties. Patients in which such regressions occurred lived for more than twenty years without recurrence of the malignant tumor.

It appears, therefore, that if we are really to come to grips with the tumor problem, we shall have to learn, as the multipotential cell has learned, how to switch the pattern of synthesis in a cell from one that makes it grow as a malignant cell to one that restores its normal or (in those instances in which extensive deletions or significant aneuploidy have occurred) at least nonmalignant state. In order to do this it would appear necessary to gain insight into such fundamental developmental processes as cellular competence, metaplasia, induction, determination, and transdetermination, all of which ultimately appear to depend for their expression on the gene action system and, more particularly, on the regulatory mechanisms that determine which of the genes in a cell are active and which are repressed. If a genuine understanding of the tumor problem were achieved and it became possible to manipulate nuclear function at will, it would provide a promising and above all a rational alternative to the rather inadequate chemotherapeutic methods that are now in use.

REFERENCES

1. Abelev, G. I., Perova, S. D., Khramkova, N. I., Postnikova, Z. A., and Irlin, I. S. *Biokhimiya* **28**, 625 (1963).
2. Abell, C. W., and Heidelberger, C. *Cancer Research* **22**, 931 (1962).
3. Abercrombie, M., and Ambrose, E. J. *Cancer Research* **22**, 525 (1962).
4. Abercrombie, M., and Heaysman, J. E. M. *Exp. Cell Research* **6**, 293 (1954).
5. Adler, H. I., Fisher, W. D., and Stapleton, G. E. *Science* **154**, 417 (1966).
6. Ahlström, C. G., and Mark, J. *Internat. J. Cancer* **1**, 51 (1966).
7. Ahuja, M. R. *Quart. Rev. Biol.* **40**, 329 (1965).
8. Aisenberg, A. C., and Morris, H. P. *Nature* **191**, 1314 (1961).
9. Aisenberg, A. C., and Morris, H. P. *Cancer Research* **23**, 566 (1963).
10. Aksenova, N. N., Bresler, V. M., Vorobyev, V. I., and Olenov, J. M. *Nature* **196**, 443 (1962).
11. Allfrey, V. G. In: *Functional Biochemistry of Cell Structures* (O. Lindberg, ed.) p. 127. Pergamon Press, Oxford, 1963. (Proc. 5th Internat. Congr. Biochemistry **2**, Moscow, 1961.)
12. Allfrey, V. G. *Canadian Cancer Research Conference* **6**, 313 (1966).
13. Allfrey, V. G. *Cancer Research* **26**, 2026 (1966).
14. Allfrey, V. G., Faulkner, R., and Mirsky, A. E. *Proc. Nat. Acad. Sci. U. S.* **51**, 786 (1964).
15. Allfrey, V. G., Littau, V. C., and Mirsky, A. E. *Proc. Nat. Acad. Sci. U. S.* **49**, 414 (1963).
16. Allfrey, V. G., and Mirsky, A. E. *Proc. Nat. Acad. Sci. U. S.* **48**, 1590 (1962).
17. Allfrey, V. G., Mirsky, A. E., and Osawa, S. *Nature* **176**, 1042 (1955).
18. Allfrey, V. G., Mirsky, A. E., and Osawa, S. *J. Gen. Physiol.* **40**, 451 (1957).
19. Ambrose, E. J. In: *The Biology of Cancer* (E. J. Ambrose and F. J. C. Roe, eds.) p. 65. Van Nostrand, London and Princeton, 1966.
20. Anders, F. *Experientia* **23**, 1 (1967).
21. Andrewes, C. H. *Lancet* **ii**, 63 and 117 (1934).
22. Askanazy, M. *Centralbl. Bakt. Parasitenk., Abt. I.* **28**, 491 (1900).
23. Bader, J. P. *Science* **149**, 757 (1965).
24. Bader, J. P. *Virology* **26**, 253 (1965).
25. Bagg, H. J. *Am. J. Cancer* **26**, 69 (1936).

26. Bakay, B., and Sorof, S. *Cancer Research* **24**, 1814 (1964).
27. Baltzer, F. *Experientia* **8**, 285 (1952).
28. Banerjee, M. R. *J. Nat. Cancer Inst.* **35**, 585 (1965).
29. Banerjee, M. R., and DeOme, K. B. *Cancer Research* **23**, 546 (1963).
30. Barr, G. C., and Butler, J. A. V. *Nature* **199**, 1170 (1963).
31. Barr, M. L. *Science* **130**, 679 (1959).
32. Barski, G. *Symp. Internat. Soc. Cell Biol.* **3**, 1 (1964).
33. Barski, G., and Belehradek, J., Jr. *Exp. Cell Research* **37**, 464 (1965).
34. Barski, G., and Cassingena, R. *J. Nat. Cancer Inst.* **30**, 865 (1963).
35. Barski, G., and Cornefert, F. *J. Nat. Cancer Inst.* **28**, 801 (1962).
36. Barski, G., Sorieul, S., and Cornefert, F. *C. r. Acad. Sci., Paris* **251**, 1825 (1960).
37. Barski, G., Sorieul, S., and Cornefert, F. *J. Nat. Cancer Inst.* **26**, 1269 (1961).
38. Barth, L. G. *Biol. Bull.* **131**, 415 (1966).
39. Baserga, R. *Cancer Research* **25**, 581 (1965).
40. Baserga, R., Estensen, R. D., and Petersen, R. O. *Proc. Nat. Acad. Sci. U. S.* **54**, 1141 (1965).
41. Bayreuther, K. *Nature* **186**, 6 (1960).
42. Beale, G. H. *Proc. Roy. Soc. London, Ser. B,* **148**, 308 (1958).
43. Beermann, W. *Chromosoma* **5**, 139 (1952).
44. Beermann, W. *Chromosoma* **12**, 1 (1961).
45. Beermann, W. In: *Cell Differentiation and Morphogenesis.* International Lecture Course, Wageningen, The Netherlands, April 26–29, 1965. p. 24. North-Holland Publ., Amsterdam, 1966.
46. Beisson, J., and Sonneborn, T. M. *Proc. Nat. Acad. Sci. U. S.* **53**, 275 (1965).
47. Benjamin, T. L. *J. Mol. Biol.* **16**, 359 (1966).
48. Berenblum, I. *Cancer Research* **1**, 807 (1941).
49. Berenblum, I., and Trainin, N. In: *Cellular Basis and Aetiology of Late Somatic Effects of Ionizing Radiation.* A symposium held in London March 27–30, 1962, under the auspices of UNESCO and the IAEA (R. J. C. Harris, ed.) p. 41. Academic Press, London, 1963.
50. Berwald, Y., and Sachs, L. *Nature* **200**, 1182 (1963).
51. Berwald, Y., and Sachs, L. *J. Nat. Cancer Inst.* **35**, 641 (1965).
52. Biemann, K., Lioret, C., Asselineau, J., Lederer, E., and Polonsky, (Mrs.) J. *Biochim. Biophys. Acta* **40**, 369 (1960).
53. Bittner, J. J. *Science* **84**, 162 (1936).
54. Bittner, J. J. *Am. J. Cancer* **35**, 90 (1939).
55. Bittner, J. J. *J. Nat. Cancer Inst.* **1**, 155 (1940).
56. Bittner, J. J. *Science* **95**, 462 (1942).
57. Black, L. M. *Proc. Am. Philos. Soc.* **88**, 132 (1944).
58. Black, L. M. *Am. J. Botany* **38**, 256 (1951).
59. Black, L. M. In: *Proceedings, Conference on Abnormal Growth in*

Plants, University of California, Berkeley, California, Nov. 5–6, 1964 (J. E. DeVay and E. E. Wilson, eds.) Final Discussion, p. 49. (Mimeo. ed.) Univ. California, 1964.

60. Black, L. M. In: *Encyclopedia of Plant Physiology* (W. Ruhland, ed.) 15/2, 236. Springer-Verlag, Berlin, Heidelberg, New York, 1965.
61. Blandau, R. J., and Young, W. C. *Am. J. Anatomy* **64**, 303 (1939).
62. Blum, H. F. *J. Nat. Cancer Inst.* **11**, 463 (1950).
63. Bonner, J., and Ts'o, P. O. P., eds. *The Nucleohistones.* 398 pp. Holden-Day, San Francisco, 1964.
64. Borek, C., and Sachs, L. *Nature* **210**, 276 (1966).
65. Borek, C., and Sachs, L. *Proc. Nat. Acad. Sci. U. S.* **56**, 1705 (1966).
66. Borrel, A. *Ztschr. Krebsforsch.* **32**, 646 (1930).
67. Boutwell, R. K. *Progr. Exp. Tumor Research* **4**, 207 (1964).
68. Boveri, T. *Anat. Anz.* **2**, 688 (1887).
69. Boveri, T. *Zellenstudien.* Heft 1–2. G. Fischer, Jena, 1887–1888.
70. Boveri, T. *Ueber mehrpolige Mitosen als Mittel zur Analyse des Zellkerns.* C. Kabitzsch, Würzburg, 1902.
71. Boveri, T. *Zellenstudien.* Heft 6. G. Fischer, Jena, 1907.
72. Boveri, T. *The Origin of Malignant Tumors.* Translated by Marcella Boveri. 119 pp. Williams and Wilkins, Baltimore, 1929.
73. Boyse, E. A., Old, L. J., Campbell, H. A., and Mashburn, L. T. *J. Exp. Med.* **125**, 17 (1967).
74. Braun, A. C. *Am. J. Botany* **30**, 674 (1943).
75. Braun, A. C. *Am. J. Botany* **34**, 234 (1947).
76. Braun, A. C. *Growth* **16**, 65 (1952).
77. Braun, A. C. *Botanical Gazette* **114**, 363 (1953).
78. Braun, A. C. *Cancer Research* **16**, 53 (1956).
79. Braun, A. C. *Symp. Soc. Exp. Biol.* **11**, 132 (1957).
80. Braun, A. C. *Proc. Nat. Acad. Sci. U. S.* **44**, 344 (1958).
81. Braun, A. C. *Proc. Nat. Acad. Sci. U. S.* **45**, 932 (1959).
82. Braun, A. C., and Laskaris, T. *Proc. Nat. Acad. Sci. U. S.* **28**, 468 (1942).
83. Braun, A. C., and Mandle, R. J. *Growth* **12**, 255 (1948).
84. Braun, A. C., and Stonier, T. *Protoplasmatologia* **10**, Heft 5a, 93 pp. (1958).
85. Braun, A. C., and White, P. R. *Phytopathology* **33**, 85 (1943).
86. Braun, A. C., and Wood, H. N. *Proc. Nat. Acad. Sci. U. S.* **48**, 1776 (1962).
87. Briggs, R., and Cassens, G. *Proc. Nat. Acad. Sci. U. S.* **55**, 1103 (1966).
88. Briggs, R., and King, T. J. *J. Morphology* **100**, 269 (1957).
89. Briggs, R., and King, T. J. In: *The Cell* (J. Brachet and A. E. Mirsky, eds.) **1**, 537. Academic Press, New York, 1959.
90. Briggs, R., and King, T. J. *Developmental Biol.* **2**, 252 (1960).

91. Briggs, R., King, T. J., and DiBerardino, M. A. In: *Symp. on Germ Cells and Earliest Stages of Development* (S. Ranzi, ed.) p. 441. Fondazione A. Baselli, Milan, 1960.
92. Brink, R. A. *Quart. Rev. Biol.* **37,** 1 (1962).
93. Brookes, P., and Lawley, P. D. *Nature* **202,** 781 (1964).
94. Broome, J. D. *Nature* **191,** 1114 (1961).
95. Brown, D. D., and Littna, E. *J. Mol. Biol.* **8,** 669 (1964).
96. Brues, A. M. *Advances in Cancer Research* **2,** 177 (1954).
97. Brues, A. M., Tracy, M. M., and Cohn, W. E. *J. Biol. Chem.* **155,** 619 (1944).
98. Bullough, W. S. In: *Cellular Control Mechanisms and Cancer* (P. Emmelot and O. Mühlbock, eds.) p. 124. Elsevier Publ., Amsterdam, London, New York, 1964.
99. Bullough, W. S. *Cancer Research* **25,** 1683 (1965).
100. Bullough, W. S., and Laurence, E. B. *Proc. Roy. Soc. London, Ser. B,* **151,** 517 (1960).
101. Bullough, W. S., and Laurence, E. B. In: *Advances in Biology of Skin* (W. Montagna and R. L. Dobson, eds.) *Carcinogenesis,* **7,** 1. Pergamon Press, New York, 1966.
102. Burch, P. R. J. *Nature* **195,** 241 (1962).
103. Burch, P. R. J. *Nature* **197,** 1042 (1963).
104. Burch, P. R. J. *Nature* **197,** 1145 (1963).
105. Burch, P. R. J. *Proc. Roy. Soc. London, Ser. B,* **162,** 223 (1965).
106. Burch, P. R. J. *Proc. Roy. Soc. London, Ser. B,* **162,** 240 (1965).
107. Burch, P. R. J. *Proc. Roy. Soc. London, Ser. B,* **162,** 263 (1965).
108. Burdette, W. J. *Cancer Research* **15,** 201 (1955).
109. Burnet, F. M. *The Clonal Selection Theory of Acquired Immunity.* 208 pp. Cambridge University Press, 1959.
109a. Busch, H. *An Introduction to the Biochemistry of the Cancer Cell.* p. 354. Academic Press, New York, 1962.
110. Busk, T., Clemmesen, J., and Nielsen, A. *British J. Cancer* **2,** 156 (1948).
111. Calame, S. *Arch. Anat. Microscop. Morphol. Exp.* **50,** 299 (1961).
112. Callan, H. G. *J. Cell Science* **1,** 85 (1966).
113. Carlsen, E. N., Trelle, G. J., and Schjeide, O. A. *Nature* **202,** 984 (1964).
114. Caro, L. G., and van Tubergen, R. P. *J. Cell Biology* **15,** 173 (1962).
115. *Chemical and Engineering News,* pp. 46–48. May 27, 1968.
116. Chevremont, M. *Bordeaux Chirurgical* **3,** 150 (1955).
117. Chuang, H. H. *Chin. J. Exp. Biology* **4,** 183 (1955).
118. Clement, A. C. *J. Exp. Zoology* **121,** 593 (1952).
119. Clement, A. C. *J. Exp. Zoology* **132,** 427 (1956).
120. Clement, A. C. *J. Exp. Zoology* **149,** 193 (1962).
121. Clever, U. *Chromosoma* **12,** 607 (1961).
122. Clever, U. *Brookhaven Symp. Biology* **18,** 242 (1965).

123. Cohen, S. *National Cancer Institute Monograph* No. **13**, pp. 13–21 (1964).

124. Cohnheim, J. F. *Vorlesungen über allgemeine Pathologie.* **1**, 622. A. Hirschwald, Berlin, 1877.

125. Collier, J. R. *Exp. Cell Research* **24**, 320 (1961).

126. Coman, D. R. *Cancer Research* **4**, 625 (1944).

127. Coman, D. R. *Cancer Research* **20**, 1202 (1960).

128. Coman, D. R., and Anderson, T. F. *Cancer Research* **15**, 541 (1955).

129. Conklin, E. G. *J. Acad. Nat. Sci. Philadelphia,* Ser. 2, **13**, 1 (1905).

130. Cook, J. W., Hewett, C. L., and Hieger, I. *J. Chem. Soc.* p. 395 (1933).

131. Coulombre, J. L., and Coulombre, A. J. *Science* **142**, 1489 (1963).

132. Craddock, C. G., Jr. *Am. J. Med.* **28**, 711 (1960).

133. Craddock, C. G. In: *Progress in Hematology* (L. M. Tocantins, ed.) **3**, 92. Grune & Stratton, New York, 1962.

134. Crick, F. H. C., Barnett, L., Brenner, S., and Watts-Tobin, R. J. *Nature* **192**, 1227 (1961).

134a. Crouse, H. V. *Proc. Nat. Acad. Sci. U. S.* **61**, 971 (1968).

135. Currie, G. A. *Lancet* **ii**, 1336 (1967).

136. Curtis, A. S. G. *J. Embryol. Exp. Morphol.* **10**, 410 (1962).

137. Curtis, H. J. *Science* **141**, 686 (1963).

138. Cushing, H., and Wolbach, S. B. *Am. J. Pathol.* **3**, 203 (1927).

139. Daniels, E. W. *Ann. New York Acad. Sci.* **78**, 662 (1959).

140. Dargeon, H. W. *J. Pediatrics* **61**, 456 (1962).

140a. Darlington, C. D., and Mather, K. *The Elements of Genetics.* 446 pp. Macmillan, New York, 1949.

141. Davidson, E. H., Haslett, G. W., Finney, R. J., Allfrey, V. G., and Mirsky, A. E. *Proc. Nat. Acad. Sci. U. S.* **54**, 696 (1965).

142. Davidson, E. H., and Mirsky, A. E. *Brookhaven Symp. Biology* **18**, 77 (1965).

143. Davidson, R. L., and Ephrussi, B. *Nature* **205**, 1170 (1965).

144. DeCarvalho, S., and Rand, H. J. *Nature* **189**, 815 (1961).

145. Defendi, V., Ephrussi, B., Koprowski, H., and Yoshida, M. C. *Proc. Nat. Acad. Sci. U. S.* **57**, 299 (1967).

146. Defendi, V., Lehman, J., and Kraemer, P. *Virology* **19**, 592 (1963).

147. de Lustig, E. S., and Lustig, L. *Rev. Soc. Argent. Biol.* **40**, 207 (1964).

148. de Terra, N. *Developmental Biol.* **10**, 269 (1964).

149. de Terra, N. *Proc. Nat. Acad. Sci. U. S.* **57**, 607 (1967).

150. Devergie, M. G. A. *Traité pratique des Maladies de la Peau.* 2nd ed. Masson, Paris, 1857.

151. DiBerardino, M. A., and King, T. J. *Developmental Biol.* **11**, 217 (1965).

152. DiBerardino, M. A., King, T. J., and McKinnell, R. G. *J. Nat. Cancer Inst.* **31**, 769 (1963).

153. DiMayorca, G. A., Eddy, B. E., Stewart, S. E., Hunter, W. S., Friend, C., and Bendich, A. *Proc. Nat. Acad. Sci. U. S.* **45**, 1805 (1959).
154. Doerfler, W. *Proc. Nat. Acad. Sci. U. S.* **60**, 636 (1968).
155. Doorenbos, J. *Proc. K. Nederl. Akad. Wetenschappen*, Ser. C, **57**, 99 (1954).
156. Dougherty, R. M., and Di Stefano, H. S. *Virology* **27**, 351 (1965).
157. Driesch, H. *Arch. Entwicklungsmech. Organismen* **7**, 65 (1898).
158. Duesberg, P. H. *Proc. Nat. Acad. Sci. U. S.* **60**, 1511 (1968).
159. Dulbecco, R. *National Cancer Institute Monograph* No. **4**, pp. 355–361 (1960).
160. Dulbecco, R. *Cancer Research* **20**, 751 (1960).
161. Dulbecco, R. *Scientific American* **216**, No. 4, 28 (1967).
162. Duran-Reynals, F. *Ann. New York Acad. Sci.* **54**, 977 (1952).
163. Duryee, W. R. *J. Franklin Inst.* **261**, 377 (1956).
164. Earle, W. R., and Nettleship, A. *J. Nat. Cancer Inst.* **4**, 213 (1943).
165. Easty, G. C. In: *The Biology of Cancer* (E. J. Ambrose and F. J. C. Roe, eds.) p. 78. Van Nostrand, London and Princeton, 1966.
166. Eddy, B. E., Borman, G. S., Berkeley, W., and Young, R. D. *Proc. Soc. Exp. Biol. Med.* **107**, 191 (1961).
167. Eddy, B. E., Borman, G. S., Grubbs, G. E., and Young, R. D. *Virology* **17**, 65 (1962).
168. Edström, J. E., and Gall, J. G. *J. Cell Biology* **19**, 279 (1963).
169. Ellermann, V., and Bang, O. *Centralbl. Bakt. Parasitenk., Abt. I, Orig.* **46**, 595 (1908).
170. Ephrussi, B. In: University of Texas M. D. Anderson Hospital and Tumor Institute, Houston, Texas. *Developmental and Metabolic Control Mechanisms and Neoplasia.* 19th Annual Symposium on Fundamental Cancer Research 1965. p. 486. Williams and Wilkins, Baltimore, 1965.
171. Ephrussi, B., and Sorieul, S. *C. r. Acad. Sci., Paris* **254**, 181 (1962).
172. Erichsen, S., Eng, J., and Morgan, H. R. *J. Exp. Med.* **114**, 435 (1961).
173. Evans, T. E. *Biochem. Biophys. Research Commun.* **22**, 678 (1966).
174. Everson, T. C., and Cole, W. H. *Spontaneous Regression of Cancer.* 560 pp. W. B. Saunders, Philadelphia and London, 1966.
175. Ewing, J. *Neoplastic Diseases.* 4th ed., rev. and enl. 1160 pp. W. B. Saunders, Philadelphia and London, 1940.
176. Faiman, C., Colwell, J. A., Ryan, R. J., Hershman, J. M., and Shields, T. W. *New England J. Med.* **277**, 1395 (1967).
177. Fankhauser, G. *Ann. New York Acad. Sci.* **49**, 684 (1948).
178. Fell, H. B., and Mellanby, E. *J. Physiology* **119**, 470 (1953).
179. Fibiger, J. *Ztschr. Krebsforsch.* **13**, 217 (1913).
180. Fieser, L. F., Fieser, M., Hershberg, E. B., Newman, M. S., Seligman, A. M., and Shear, M. *J. Am. J. Cancer* **29**, 260 (1937).
181. Flickinger, R. A., and Stone, G. *Exp. Cell Research* **21**, 541 (1960).

182. Fogel, M., and Sachs, L. *Developmental Biol.* 10, 411 (1964).
183. Fogel, M., and Sachs, L. *Exp. Cell Research* 34, 448 (1964).
184. Foley, G. E., and Drolet, B. P. *Cancer Research* 24, 1461 (1964).
185. Ford, E. B. *Genetics for Medical Students.* 4th ed. London, 1956.
186. Fosket, D. E. *Proc. Nat. Acad. Sci. U. S.* 59, 1089 (1968).
187. Foulds, L. In: *Cellular Control Mechanisms and Cancer* (P. Emmelot and O. Mühlbock, eds.) p. 242. Elsevier Publ., Amsterdam, 1964.
188. Frank, H., and Renner, O. *Planta* 47, 105 (1956).
189. Fried, M. *Proc. Nat. Acad. Sci. U. S.* 53, 486 (1965).
190. Fujinaga, K., and Green, M. *Proc. Nat. Acad. Sci. U. S.* 55, 1567 (1966).
191. Gall, J. G. In: *Cytodifferentiation and Macromolecular Synthesis* (M. Locke, ed.) p. 119. Academic Press, New York and London, 1963.
192. Gall, J. G., and Callan, H. G. *Proc. Nat. Acad. Sci. U. S.* 48, 562 (1962).
193. Gallera, J. *Arch. Entwicklungsmech. Organismen* 146, 21 (1952).
194. Garriga, S., and Crosby, W. H. *Blood* 14, 1008 (1959).
195. Gautheret, R. J. *C. r. Soc. Biol.* 140, 169 (1946).
196. Gelfant, S. *Exp. Cell Research* 26, 395 (1962).
197. Gelfant, S. *Symp. Internat. Soc. Cell Biology* 2, 229 (1963).
198. Gelfant, S. In: *Methods in Cell Physiology* (D. M. Prescott, ed.) 2, 359. Academic Press, New York, 1966.
199. Gershon, D., and Sachs, L. *Nature* 198, 912 (1963).
200. Gey, G. O. *Cancer Research* 1, 737 (1941).
201. Gey, G. O. *The Harvey Lectures* 50 (*1954–1955*), 154 (1956).
202. Girardi, A. J., Sweet, B. H., Slotnick, V. B., and Hilleman, M. R. *Proc. Soc. Exp. Biol. Med.* 109, 649 (1962).
203. Gilbert, W., and Müller-Hill, B. *Proc. Nat. Acad. Sci. U. S.* 56, 1891 (1966).
204. Gold, M., and Helleiner, C. W. *Biochim. Biophys. Acta* 80, 193 (1964).
205. Gold, P., and Freedman, S. O. *J. Exp. Med.* 122, 467 (1965).
206. Goldé, A., and Latarjet, R. *C. r. Acad. Sci., Paris, Ser. D,* 262, 420 (1966).
207. Goldstein, M. N., Burdman, J. A., and Journey, L. J. *J. Nat. Cancer Inst.* 32, 165 (1964).
208. Goodman, R. M., Goidl, J., and Richart, R. M. *Proc. Nat. Acad. Sci. U. S.* 58, 553 (1967).
209. Gorer, P. A. In: *Clinical Genetics* (A. Sorsby, ed.) p. 558. Butterworth, London, 1953.
210. Graham, C. F., Arms, K., and Gurdon, J. B. *Developmental Biol.* 14, 349 (1966).
211. Granboulan, N., and Granboulan, P. *Exp. Cell Research* 38, 604 (1965).
212. Greene, H. S. N. *J. Exp. Med.* 71, 305 (1940).

213. Greenstein, J. P. *Cancer Research* **16**, 641 (1956).
214. Grobstein, C. *Exp. Cell Research* **10**, 424 (1956).
215. Grobstein, C. In: *The Cell* (J. Brachet and A. E. Mirsky, eds.), **1**, 437. Academic Press, New York, 1959.
216. Gross, L. *Proc. Soc. Exp. Biol. Med.* **76**, 27 (1951).
217. Gross, L. *Proc. Soc. Exp. Biol. Med.* **83**, 414 (1953).
218. Gross, L. *Proc. Soc. Exp. Biol. Med.* **100**, 102 (1959).
219. Gurdon, J. B. *Proc. Nat. Acad. Sci. U. S.* **58**, 545 (1967).
220. Gurdon, J. B., and Uehlinger, V. *Nature* **210**, 1240 (1966).
221. Habel, K. *Proc. Soc. Exp. Biol. Med.* **106**, 722 (1961).
222. Hadorn, E. *Brookhaven Symp. Biol.* **18**, 148 (1965).
223. Hadorn, E., Bertani, G., and Gallera, J. *Arch. Entwicklungsmech. Organismen* **144**, 31 (1949).
224. Haggard, H. W. *Bull. New York Acad. Med.*, ser. 2, **14**, 183 (1938).
225. Halberstaedter, L., Doljanski, L., and Tenenbaum, E. *Brit. J. Exp. Path.* **22**, 179 (1941).
226. Hamperl, H. *Wiener klin. Wochenschrift* **69**, 201 (1957).
227. Hanau, A. N. *Arch. klin. Chirurgie* **39**, 678 (1889).
228. Harris, H. *J. Cell Science* **2**, 23 (1967).
229. Hauschka, T. S. *Cancer Research* **21**, 957 (1961).
230. Hauschka, T. S., and Levan, A. *J. Nat. Cancer Inst.* **21**, 77 (1958).
231. Hauser, G. *Beitr. path. Anat. u. Path., Jena* **33**, 1 (1903).
232. Häussler, G. *Klin. Wochenschrift* **7**, 1561 (1928).
232a. Hay, E. D. In: *The Stability of the Differentiated State* (H. Ursprung, ed.) p. 85. Springer-Verlag, Berlin and New York, 1968. (Results and Problems in Cell Differentiation, v. 1.)
233. Hayflick, L., and Moorhead, P. S. *Exp. Cell Research* **25**, 585 (1961).
234. Hegner, R. W. *J. Morphology* **25**, 375 (1914).
235. Helgeson, J. P. *Science* **161**, 974 (1968).
236. Heston, W. E. *British J. Cancer* **2**, 87 (1948).
237. Heston, W. E., Deringer, M. K., Dunn, T. B., and Levillain, W. D. *J. Nat. Cancer Inst.* **10**, 1139 (1950).
238. Hieger, I. *Biochem. J.* **24**, 505 (1930).
239. Hieger, I. *Carcinogenesis.* 138 pp. Academic Press, London and New York, 1961.
240. Hindley, J. *Biochem. Biophys. Research Commun.* **12**, 175 (1963).
241. Holley, R. W., and Kiernan, J. A. *Proc. Nat. Acad. Sci. U. S.* **60**, 300 (1968).
242. Holtfreter, J. *Arch. Entwicklungsmech. Organismen* **138**, 163 (1938).
243. Holtfreter, J. *Ann. New York Acad. Sci.* **49**, 709 (1948).
243a. Hondius Boldingh, W., and Laurence, E. B. *European J. Biochemistry* **5**, 191 (1968).
244. Hotta, Y., and Stern, H. *Proc. Nat. Acad. Sci. U. S.* **49**, 648 (1963).
245. Hotta, Y., and Stern, H. *Proc. Nat. Acad. Sci. U. S.* **49**, 861 (1963).

246. Hotta, Y., and Stern, H. *J. Cell Biology* **16,** 259 (1963).
247. Hotta, Y., and Stern, H. *J. Cell Biology* **19,** 45 (1963).
248. Hotta, Y., and Stern, H. *J. Cell Biology* **25,** no. 3, pt. 2, p. 99 (1965).
249. Hsu, T. C. *Internat. Rev. Cytology* **12,** 69 (1961).
250. Huang, R. C., and Bonner, J. *Proc. Nat. Acad. Sci. U. S.* **48,** 1216 (1962).
251. Huang, R. C., and Bonner, J. *Proc. Nat. Acad. Sci. U. S.* **54,** 960 (1965).
252. Huebner, R. J., Armstrong, D., Okuyan, M., Sarma, P. S., and Turner, H. C. *Proc. Nat. Acad. Sci. U. S.* **51,** 742 (1964).
253. Huebner, R. J., Rowe, W. P., Turner, H. C., and Lane, W. T. *Proc. Nat. Acad. Sci. U. S.* **50,** 379 (1963).
254. Huettner, A. F. *J. Morphology* **37,** 385 (1923).
255. Hurwitz, J., Evans, A., Babinet, C., and Skalka, A. *Cold Spring Harbor Symp. Quant. Biol.* **28,** 59 (1963).
256. Inoué, S., and Sato, H. *J. Gen. Physiol.* **50,** no. 6, pt. 2, p. 259 (1967).
257. Izawa, M., Allfrey, V. G., and Mirsky, A. E. *Proc. Nat. Acad. Sci. U. S.* **49,** 544 (1963).
258. Izawa, M., Allfrey, V. G., and Mirsky, A. E. *Proc. Nat. Acad. Sci. U. S.* **50,** 811 (1963).
259. Jablonski, J. R., and Skoog, F. *Physiol. Plantarum* **7,** 16 (1954).
260. Jacob, F., Brenner, S., and Cuzin, F. *Cold Spring Harbor Symp. Quant. Biol.* **28,** 329 (1963).
261. Jacob, F., and Monod, J. *J. Mol. Biol.* **3,** 318 (1961).
262. Jacob, F., and Monod, J. In: *Cytodifferentiation and Macromolecular Synthesis* (M. Locke, ed.) p. 30. Academic Press, New York and London, 1963.
263. Jacoby, F., Trowell, O. A., and Willmer, E. N. *J. Exp. Biol.* **14,** 255 (1937).
264. Jensen, C. O. *Hospitalstidende* **11,** 549 and 581 (1903).
265. Jensen, C. O. *Centralbl. Bakt. Parasitenk., Abt. I, Orig.* **34,** 28 and 122 (1903).
266. Jensen, C. O. *Ztschr. Krebsforsch.* **7,** 45 (1909).
267. Jensen, C. O. *Von echten Geschwülsten bei Pflanzen.* Deuxième Conférence Internationale pour l'Étude du Cancer, tenue a Paris du 1er au 5 octobre 1910. p. 243. Félix Alcan, Éditeur, Paris, 1910.
268. Jinks, J. L. *Extrachromosomal Inheritance.* 177 pp. Prentice-Hall, Englewood Cliffs, N. J., 1964.
269. Johnson, I. S. *Cancer Research* **18,** 367 (1958).
270. Jollos, V. *Arch. Protistenkunde* **43,** 1 (1921).
271. Kane, R. E. *J. Cell Biology* **32,** 243 (1967).
272. Kark, W. *A Synopsis of Cancer. Genesis and Biology.* 280 pp. John Wright and Sons, Bristol, 1966.
273. Karlson, P. In: *Induktion und Morphogenese,* p. 101. Springer-Verlag, Berlin, 1963. (Gesell. Physiol. Chemie, 1962, Colloq. v. 13.)

274. Kehr, A. E., and Smith, H. H. *Cornell Univ. Agr. Exp. Station Memoir* **311**, 19 pp. 1952.
275. Kehr, A. E., and Smith, H. H. *Brookhaven Symp. Biol.* **6**, 55 (1954).
276. Kemp, T. *British J. Cancer* **2**, 144 (1948).
277. Kende, H., and Tavares, J. E. *Plant Physiol.* **43**, 1244 (1968).
278. Kennaway, E. L. *Biochem. J.* **24**, 497 (1930).
279. Kennaway, E. L., and Hieger, I. *British Med. J.* **1**, 1044 (1930).
280. Kidd, J. G. *J. Exp. Med.* **98**, 565 (1953).
281. Kidson, C., and Kirby, K. S. *Nature* **203**, 599 (1964).
282. Kidson, C., and Kirby, K. S. *Cancer Research* **24**, 1604 (1964).
283. Kidson, C., and Kirby, K. S. *Cancer Research* **25**, 472 (1965).
284. Kiefer, B., Sakai, H., Solari, A. J., and Mazia, D. *J. Mol. Biol.* **20**, 75 (1966).
285. Kimball, R. F., and Prescott, D. M. *J. Protozoology* **9**, 88 (1962).
286. King, T. J., and Briggs, R. *J. Embryol. Exp. Morphol.* **2**, 73 (1954).
287. King, T. J., and Briggs, R. *Proc. Nat. Acad. Sci. U. S.* **41**, 321 (1955).
288. King, T. J., and Briggs, R. *Cold Spring Harbor Symp. Quant. Biol.* **21**, 271 (1956).
289. Klein, G., and Klein, E. *Symp. Soc. Exp. Biol.* **11**, 305 (1957).
290. Kleinenberg, H. E., Neufach, S. A., and Schabad, L. M. *Cancer Research* **1**, 853 (1941).
291. Kleinsmith, L. J., Allfrey, V. G., and Mirsky, A. E. *Proc. Nat. Acad. Sci. U. S.* **55**, 1182 (1966).
292. Kleinsmith, L. J., and Pierce, G. B., Jr. *Cancer Research* **24**, 1544 (1964).
293. Koller, P. C. *Symp. Soc. Exp. Biol.* **1**, 270 (1947).
294. Koller, P. C. In: University of Texas M. D. Anderson Hospital and Tumor Institute, Houston, Texas. *Cell Physiology of Neoplasia.* Symposium on Fundamental Cancer Research 1960. p. 9. Univ. Texas Press, Austin, 1960.
295. Koop, C. E., Kiesewetter, W. B., and Horn, R. C., Jr. *Surgery* **38**, 272 (1955).
296. Koprowski, H., Jensen, F. C., and Steplewski, Z. *Proc. Nat. Acad. Sci. U. S.* **58**, 127 (1967).
297. Kranz, G. *Flora (Jena)* **125**, 289 (1931).
298. Kroeger, H. *Nature* **200**, 1234 (1963).
299. Langan, T. A., and Smith, L. *NIH Information Exchange Group, Scientific Memo* No. 113, 1965.
300. Latarjet, R. *Cancer Research* **20**, 807 (1960).
301. Ledbetter, M. C., and Porter, K. R. *J. Cell Biology* **19**, 239 (1963).
302. Levan, A. *Hereditas* **57**, 343 (1967).
303. Levan, A., and Biesele, J. J. *Ann. New York Acad. Sci.* **71**, 1022 (1958).
304. Levander, G. *Surg. Gynecol. Obstet.* **67**, 705 (1938).
305. Levi-Montalcini, R. *Ann. New York Acad. Sci.* **118**, 149 (1964).

306. Lieberman, I., Abrams, R., Hunt, N., and Ove, P. *J. Biol. Chem.* **238**, 3955 (1963).
307. Lieberman, M., and Kaplan, H. S. *Science* **130**, 387 (1959).
308. Lillie, F. R. *J. Exp. Zoology* **3**, 153 (1906).
309. Lima-de-Faria, A., Reitalu, J., and Bergman, S. *Hereditas* **47**, 695 (1961).
310. Limasset, P., and Gautheret, R. *C. r. Acad. Sci., Paris* **230**, 2043 (1950).
311. Lioret, C. *Bull. Soc. Franç. Physiol. Veg.* **2**, 76 (1956).
312. Littau, V. C., Allfrey, V. G., Frenster, J. H., and Mirsky, A. E. *Proc. Nat. Acad. Sci. U. S.* **52**, 93 (1964).
313. Littau, V. C., and Black, L. M. *Am. J. Botany* **39**, 191 (1952).
314. Littau, V. C., Burdick, C. J., Allfrey, V. G., and Mirsky, A. E. *Proc. Nat. Acad. Sci. U. S.* **54**, 1204 (1965).
315. Little, C. C. *Proc. Nat. Acad. Sci. U. S.* **25**, 452 (1939).
316. Little, C. C. *Biol. Rev. Cambridge Philos. Soc.* **22**, 315 (1947).
317. Loeb, L. *J. Med. Research* n.s., **1**, 28 (1901).
318. Loeb, L. *Acta Unio Internationalis contra Cancrum* **2**, 148 (1937).
319. Loeb, L. *The Biological Basis of Individuality.* 711 pp. C. C. Thomas, Springfield, Ill., 1945.
320. Loewenstein, W. R., and Kanno, Y. *J. Cell Biology* **33**, 225 (1967).
321. Loewenstein, W. R., and Penn, R. D. *J. Cell Biology* **33**, 235 (1967).
322. Lubs, H. A., Jr., and Clark, R. *New England J. Med.* **268**, 907 (1963).
323. Lucké, B. *Am. J. Cancer* **20**, 352 (1934).
324. Lucké, B. *J. Exp. Med.* **68**, 457 (1938).
325. Lunger, P. D. *Virology* **24**, 138 (1964).
326. Lynch, C. J. *J. Exp. Med.* **39**, 481 (1924).
327. Lynch, H. T. *Hereditary Factors in Carcinoma.* 186 pp. Springer, New York, 1967. (Recent Results in Cancer Research, v. 12.)
328. Lyon, M. F. *Am. J. Human Genetics* **14**, 135 (1962).
329. MacKenzie, I., and Rous, P. *J. Exp. Med.* **73**, 391 (1941).
330. Macpherson, I. *Science* **148**, 1731 (1965).
331. Magee, P. N., and Farber, E. *Biochem. J.* **83**, 114 (1962).
332. Maisel, H., and Harmison, C. *J. Embryol. Exp. Morph.* **11**, 483 (1963).
333. Makino, S. *Chromosoma* **4**, 649 (1952).
334. Makino, S. *Ann. New York Acad. Sci.* **63**, 818 (1956).
335. Makino, S., and Kanô, K. *J. Nat. Cancer Inst.* **15**, 1165 (1955).
336. Manaker, R. A., and Groupé, V. *Virology* **2**, 838 (1956).
337. Marie, P., Clunet, J., and Raulot-Lapointe, G. *Bull. Assoc. Franç. Etude Cancer* **3**, 404 (1910).
338. Marie, P., Clunet, J., and Raulot-Lapointe, G. *Bull. Assoc. Franç. Etude Cancer* **3**, 166 (1911).
339. Marie, P., Clunet, J., and Raulot-Lapointe, G. *Bull. Assoc. Franç. Etude Cancer* **5**, 125 (1912).

340. Marks, L. J., Russfield, A. B., and Rosenbaum, D. L. *J. Am. Med. Assoc.* **183**, no. 2, p. 115 (1963).
341. Marroquin, F., and Farber, E. *Cancer Research* **25**, 1262 (1965).
342. Marsh, M. C. *J. Cancer Research* **13**, 313 (1929).
343. Martin, C. M., Magnusson, S., Goscienski, P. J., and Hansen, G. F. *Science* **134**, 1985 (1961).
344. Maxwell, T. *Lancet* **i**, 152 (1879).
345. Mazia, D. In: *The Cell* (J. Brachet and A. E. Mirsky, eds.) **3**, 77. Academic Press, New York, 1961.
346. Mazia, D., and Dan, K. *Proc. Nat. Acad. Sci. U. S.* **38**, 826 (1952).
347. Mazia, D., and Roslansky, J. D. *Protoplasma* **46**, 528 (1956).
348. McCarthy, B. J., and Hoyer, B. H. *Proc. Nat. Acad. Sci. U. S.* **52**, 915 (1964).
349. McCreight, C. E., and Andrew, W. *Anat. Record* **125**, 761 (1956).
350. McFarland, J., and Meade, T. S. *Am. J. Med. Sciences* **184**, 66 (1932).
351. McIntosh, J., and Selbie, F. R. *British J. Exp. Path.* **20**, 49 (1939).
352. McKinnell, R. G. *Am. Zoologist* **2**, 430 (1962).
353. Ménagé, A., and Morel, G. *C. r. Acad. Sci., Paris* **259**, 4795 (1964).
354. Ménagé, A., and Morel, G. *C. r. Acad. Sci., Paris* **261**, 2001 (1965).
355. Metz, C. W. *Am. Naturalist* **72**, 485 (1938).
356. Michalowsky, I. *Arch. path. Anat. Physiol.* **267**, 27 (1928); **274**, 319 (1929).
357. Miller, E. C. *Cancer Research* **11**, 100 (1951).
358. Miller, E. C., and Miller, J. A. *Cancer Research* **7**, 468 (1947).
359. Miller, E. C., and Miller, J. A. *Pharmacol. Rev.* **18**, 805 (1966).
360. Miller, O. L. *J. Cell Biology* **23**, 109A (1964).
361. Mirsky, A. E., and Ris, H. *Nature* **163**, 666 (1949).
362. Mizell, M. *Am. Zoologist* **5**, 215 (1965).
363. Monod, J., and Jacob, F. *Cold Spring Harbor Symp. Quant. Biol.* **26**, 389 (1961).
364. Moorhead, P. S., and Saksela, E. *J. Cell. Comp. Physiol.* **62**, 57 (1963).
365. Mueller, G. C. *Exp. Cell Research Suppl.* **9**, 144 (1963).
366. Mueller, G. C., Kajiwara, K., Stubblefield, E., and Rueckert, R. R. *Cancer Research* **22**, 1084 (1962).
367. Müller, J. *Ueber den feineren Bau und die Formen der krankhaften Geschwülste.* Lief. 1. G. Reimer, Berlin, 1838.
368. Näf, U. *Growth* **22**, 167 (1958).
369. Nakas, M., Higashino, S., and Loewenstein, W. R. *Science* **151**, 89 (1966).
370. Needham, J. *Proc. Roy. Soc. Med.* **29**, 1577 (1936).
371. Needham, J. *Biochemistry and Morphogenesis.* 785 pp. University Press, Cambridge, 1942.
372. Nettleship, A., and Earle, W. R. *J. Nat. Cancer Inst.* **4**, 229 (1943).
373. Nichols, W. W. *Hereditas* **50**, 53 (1963).

374. Nichols, W. W., Levan, A., and Heneen, W. K. *Hereditas* **57**, 365 (1967).

375. Nieuwkoop, P. D. *Acta Embryol. Morphol. Exp.* **2**, 13 (1958).

376. Niu, M. C. *Science* **131**, 1321 (1960).

377. Niu, M. C., Cordova, C. C., and Niu, L. C. *Proc. Nat. Acad. Sci. U. S.* **47**, 1689 (1961).

378. Niu, M. C., and Twitty, V. C. *Proc. Nat. Acad. Sci. U. S.* **39**, 985 (1953).

379. Nordling, C. O. *British J. Cancer* **7**, 68 (1953).

380. Nöthiger, R. *Arch. Entwicklungsmech. Organismen* **155**, 269 (1964).

381. Novikoff, A. B. *Biol. Bull.* **74**, 211 (1938).

382. Nowell, P. C., and Hungerford, D. A. *J. Nat. Cancer Inst.* **27**, 1013 (1961).

383. Nowell, P. C., and Hungerford, D. A. *Ann. New York Acad. Sci.* **113**, 654 (1964).

384. Oberling, C. *The Riddle of Cancer*. Translated by William H. Woglom. 196 pp. Yale Univ. Press, New Haven, 1944.

385. Oberling, C., and Guérin, M. *Bull. Assoc. Franç. Etude Cancer* **37**, 5 (1950).

386. Oettgen, H. F., Old, L. J., Boyse, E. A., Campbell, H. A., Philips, F. S., Clarkson, B. D., Tallal, L., Leeper, R. D., Schwartz, M. K., and Kim, J. H. *Cancer Research* **27**, 2619 (1967).

387. Old, L. J., Boyse, E. A., Campbell, H. A., Brodey, R. S., Fidler, J., and Teller, J. D. *Cancer* **20**, 1066 (1967).

388. Olson, R. E. *Science* **145**, 926 (1964).

389. Parsons, J. A. *J. Cell Biology* **25**, 641 (1965).

390. Pavan, C. *Brookhaven Symp. Biol.* **18**, 222 (1965).

391. Pelling, C. *Chromosoma* **15**, 71 (1964).

392. Penn, R. D. *J. Cell Biology* **29**, 171 (1966).

393. Pierce, G. B., Jr., Dixon, F. J., Jr., and Verney, E. L. *Laboratory Investigation* **9**, 583 (1960).

394. Pitot, H. C. *Ann. Rev. Biochem.* **35**, pt. 1, p. 335 (1966).

395. Pitot, H. C., and Cho, Y. S. *Progr. Exp. Tumor Research* **7**, 158 (1965).

396. Pitot, H. C., and Heidelberger, C. *Cancer Research* **23**, 1694 (1963).

397. Pogo, B. G. T., Allfrey, V. G., and Mirsky, A. E. *Proc. Nat. Acad. Sci. U. S.* **55**, 805 (1966).

398. Politzer, G. *Arch. Entwicklungsmech. Organismen* **147**, 547 (1955).

399. Pollack, R. E., Green, H., and Todaro, G. J. *Proc. Nat. Acad. Sci. U. S.* **60**, 126 (1968).

400. Pott, P. *Chirurgical Observations Relative to the Cataract, the Polypus of the Nose, the Cancer of the Scrotum, the Different Kinds of Ruptures, and the Mortification of the Toes and Feet.* 208 pp. Hawes, London, 1775.

401. Potter, V. R. *Enzymes, Growth and Cancer.* C. C. Thomas, 1950.
402. Potter, V. R. *Fed. Proc.* **17**, 691 (1958).
403. Potter, V. R. *Cancer Research* **24**, 1085 (1964).
403a. Potter, V. R. In: *Cellular Control Mechanisms and Cancer* (P. Emmelot and O. Mühlbock, eds.) p. 190. Elsevier Publ., Amsterdam, London, New York, 1964.
404. Prescott, D. M. *National Cancer Institute Monograph* No. **14**, p. 57. Internat. Symp., 1963. National Cancer Inst., Bethesda, Md., 1964.
405. Prescott, D. M., and Goldstein, L. *Science* **155**, 469 (1967).
406. Prince, A. M. *Virology* **11**, 400 (1960).
407. Prince, A. M. *Virology* **18**, 524 (1962).
408. Prince, A. M., and Adams, W. R. *Virology* **30**, 151 (1966).
409. Puck, T. T., Waldren, C. A., and Jones, C. *Proc. Nat. Acad. Sci. U. S.* **59**, 192 (1968).
409a. Rabinowitz, Z., and Sachs, L. *Nature* **220**, 1203 (1968).
410. Rehn, L. *Arch. klin. Chirurgie* **50**, 588 (1895).
411. Reyer, R. W. *Quart. Rev. Biol.* **29**, 1 (1954).
412. Reyss-Brion, M. *J. Embryol. Exp. Morphol.* **11**, 649 (1963).
413. Reyss-Brion, M. *Arch. Anat. Microscop. Morphol. Exp.* **53**, 397 (1964).
414. Ribbert, [M. W.] H. *Das Karzinom des Menschen, sein Bau, sein Wachstum, seine Entstehung.* 526 pp. F. Cohen, Bonn, 1911.
415. Robbins, W. J. *Am. J. Botany* **44**, 743 (1957).
416. Robbins, W. J. *Am. J. Botany* **47**, 485 (1960).
417. Robert, M., and Kroeger, H. *Experientia* **21**, 326 (1965).
418. Rose, S. M., and Wallingford, H. M. *Science* **107**, 457 (1948).
419. Roth, J. S. *Nature* **207**, 599 (1965).
420. Rothfels, K. H., Kupelwieser, E. B., and Parker, R. C. *Canadian Cancer Research Conference* **5**, 191 (1963).
421. Rous, P. *J. Exp. Med.* **12**, 696 (1910).
422. Rous, P. *J. Am. Med. Assoc.* **55**, 1805 (1910).
423. Rous, P. *The Harvey Lectures* **31** (*1935–1936*), 74 (1936).
424. Rous, P. *Cancer Research* **20**, 672 (1960).
425. Rous, P. *Cancer Research* **20**, 707 (1960).
426. Rous, P., and Beard, J. W. *J. Exp. Med.* **62**, 523 (1935).
427. Rous, P., and Friedewald, W. F. *J. Exp. Med.* **79**, 511 (1944).
428. Rous, P., and Kidd, J. G. *J. Exp. Med.* **73**, 365 (1941).
429. Rous, P., Murphy, J. B., and Tytler, W. H. *J. Am. Med. Assoc.* **59**, 1793 (1912).
430. Rubin, H. *Ann. New York Acad. Sci.* **68**, 459 (1957).
431. Rubin, H. In: *Virus Growth and Variation* (A. Isaacs and B. W. Lacey, eds.) p. 171. University Press, Cambridge, 1959.
432. Rubin, H. In: *Major Problems in Developmental Biology* (M. Locke, ed.) p. 315. Academic Press, New York and London, 1966.
433. Rubin, H., and Temin, H. M. *Fed. Proc.* **17**, 994 (1958).

434. Rytömaa, T., and Kiviniemi, K. *Proc. XIVth Scand. Congr. Pathol. Microbiol.*, p. 169. Universitetsforlaget, Oslo, 1964.

435. Rytömaa, T., and Kiviniemi, K. *Cell and Tissue Kinetics* **1**, 329 and 341 (1968).

436. Saetren, H. *Exp. Cell Research* **11**, 229 (1956).

437. Saetren, H. *Acta Chem. Scand.* **17**, 889 (1963).

438. Sager, R., and Ramanis, Z. *Proc. Nat. Acad. Sci. U. S.* **50**, 260 (1963).

439. Sakai, H. *Biochim. Biophys. Acta* **112**, 132 (1966).

440. Salb, J. M., and Marcus, P. I. *Proc. Nat. Acad. Sci. U. S.* **54**, 1353 (1965).

441. Sambrook, J., Westphal, H., Srinivasan, P. R., and Dulbecco, R. *Proc. Nat. Acad. Sci. U. S.* **60**, 1288 (1968).

442. Sanford, K. K., Earle, W. R., Shelton, E., Schilling, E. L., Duchesne, E. M., Likely, G. D., and Becker, M. M. *J. Nat. Cancer Inst.* **11**, 351 (1950).

─443. Sanford, K. K., Likely, G. D., Bryan, W. R., and Earle, W. R. *J. Nat. Cancer Inst.* **12**, 1317 (1952).

444. Scaletta, L. J., and Ephrussi, B. *Nature* **205**, 1169 (1965).

445. Schabad, L. C. r. *Soc. Biol.* **124**, 213 (1937).

446. Schabad, L. M. C. r. *Soc. Biol.* **126**, 1180 (1937).

447. Schwalbe, E. *Die Morphologie und Missbildungen des Menschen und der Tiere.* II. Teil. Jena, 1907.

448. Seilern-Aspang, F., and Kratochwil, K. *J. Embryol. Exp. Morphol.* **10**, 337 (1962).

449. Seilern-Aspang, F., and Kratochwil, K. *Wiener klin. Wochenschrift* **75**, 337 (1963).

450. Seitz, E. W., and Hochster, R. M. *Canadian J. Botany* **42**, 999 (1964).

451. Shope, R. E. *J. Exp. Med.* **56**, 803 (1932).

452. Shope, R. E. *J. Exp. Med.* **58**, 607 (1933).

453. Silagi, S. *Cancer Research* **27**, 1953 (1967).

453a. Simard, A., Cousineau, G., and Daoust, R. *J. Nat. Cancer Inst.* **41**, 1257 (1968).

454. Sjögren, H. O., Hellström, I., and Klein, G. *Cancer Research* **21**, 329 (1961).

455. Skoog, F. *Am. J. Botany* **31**, 19 (1944).

456. Skoog, F., and Miller, C. O. *Symp. Soc. Exp. Biol.* **11**, 118 (1957).

457. Slizynski, B. M. *J. Genetics* **50**, 77 (1950).

458. Slye, M. *Ztschr. Krebsforsch.* **13**, 500 (1913).

459. Slye, M. *J. Med. Research* **30** (n.s. **25**), 281 (1914).

460. Slye, M. *J. Med. Research* **32** (n.s. **27**), 159 (1915).

461. Smith, E. F., and Townsend, C. O. *Science* **25**, 671 (1907).

462. Smith, H. H. *Ann. New York Acad. Sci.* **71**, 1163 (1958).

463. Smith, P. D., Koenig, P. B., and Lucchesi, J. C. *Nature* **217**, 1286 (1968).

464. Snyder, L. H. In: *Genetics, Medicine, and Man.* H. J. Muller, C. C. Little, and L. H. Snyder. p. 91. London, 1947.

465. Sonneborn, T. M. *Perspectives in Virology* **2**, 5 (1961).

466. Sonneborn, T. M. In: *The Nature of Biological Diversity* (J. M. Allen, ed.) p. 165. McGraw-Hill, New York, 1963.

467. Sonneborn, T. M. In: *The Scientific Endeavor. Centennial Celebration of the National Academy of Sciences.* p. 217. Rockefeller Institute Press, New York, 1965.

468. Sonnenberg, B. P., and Zubay, G. *Proc. Nat. Acad. Sci. U. S.* **54**, 415 (1965).

469. Sorieul, S., and Ephrussi, B. *Nature* **190**, 653 (1961).

470. Sorof, S., Cohen, P. P., Miller, E. C., and Miller, J. A. *Cancer Research* **11**, 383 (1951).

471. Sorof, S., Young, E. M., McCue, M. M., and Fetterman, P. L. *Cancer Research* **23**, 864 (1963).

472. Sparrow, A. H., and Gunckel, J. E. In: *Progress in Radiobiology.* p. 485. Oliver and Boyd, Edinburgh and London, 1956.

473. Sparrow, A. H., Gunckel, J. E., Schairer, L. A., and Hagen, G. L. *Am. J. Botany* **43**, 377 (1956).

474. Spemann, H. *Arch. Entwicklungsmech. Organismen* **43**, 448 (1918).

475. Spemann, H., and Mangold, H. *Arch. mikrosk. Anat. u. Entwicklungsmech.* **100**, 599 (1924).

476. Srb, A. M. In: *Reproduction: Molecular, Subcellular, and Cellular* (M. Locke, ed.) p. 191. Academic Press, New York and London, 1965.

476a. Stedman, E., and Stedman, E. *Philos. Trans. Royal Soc. London,* Ser. B, **235**, 565 (1951).

477. Stephens, R. E. *J. Cell Biology* **32**, 255 (1967).

478. Stern, H. *Ann. New York Acad. Sci.* **90**, 440 (1960).

479. Stern, H. *Ann. Rev. Plant Physiol.* **17**, 345 (1966).

480. Stevens, D. F. *Exp. Cell Research* **25**, 654 (1961).

481. Stevens, D. F. *Exp. Cell Research* **41**, 492 (1966).

482. Stevens, D., and Schwenk, E. *Experientia* **15**, 470 (1959).

483. Steward, F. C., Mapes, M. O., Kent, A. E., and Holsten, R. D. *Science* **143**, 20 (1964).

484. Stewart, S. E. *Anat. Record* **117**, 532 (1953).

485. Stewart, S. E., Eddy, B. E., and Borgese, N. *J. Nat. Cancer Inst.* **20**, 1223 (1958).

486. Stich, H. F., and Steele, H. D. *J. Nat. Cancer Inst.* **28**, 1207 (1962).

487. Stoker, M. *Nature* **200**, 756 (1963).

488. Stoker, M. *Virology* **24**, 165 (1964).

489. Stoker, M. *Nature* **218**, 234 (1968).

490. Stone, L. S. *Anat. Record* **106**, 89 (1950).

491. Stone, L. S. *J. Exp. Zoology* **113**, 9 (1950).

492. Stone, L. S. *J. Exp. Zoology* **127**, 463 (1954).

493. Stone, L. S. *Anat. Record* **120**, 599 (1954).

494. Stone, L. S. *Anat. Record* **131**, 151 (1958).

495. Stoutemyer, V. T., and Britt, O. K. *Nature* **199**, 397 (1963).

496. Strasburger, E. *Histologische Beiträge*, Heft VI. G. Fischer, Jena, 1900.

497. Strong, L. C. *Cancer Research* **2**, 531 (1942).

498. Stubblefield, E., and Mueller, G. C. *Cancer Research* **22**, 1091 (1962).

499. Sugiyama, T., Kurita, Y., and Nishizuka, Y. *Science* **158**, 1058 (1967).

500. Swann, M. M. *Cancer Research* **17**, 727 (1957).

501. Swann, M. M. *Cancer Research* **18**, 1118 (1958).

502. Sweet, B. H., and Hilleman, M. R. *Proc. Soc. Exp. Biol. Med.* **105**, 420 (1960).

503. Szent-Györgyi, A. *Perspectives in Biol. Med.* **7**, 279 (1964).

504. Tanaka, S., and Southam, C. M. *J. Nat. Cancer Inst.* **34**, 441 (1965).

505. Taylor, J. H. *Internat. Rev. Cytology* **13**, 39 (1962).

506. Temin, H. M. *Virology* **20**, 577 (1963).

507. Temin, H. M. *Proc. Nat. Acad. Sci. U. S.* **52**, 323 (1964).

508. Temin, H. M. *Virology* **23**, 486 (1964).

509. Temin, H. M. *J. Nat. Cancer Inst.* **35**, 679 (1965).

510. Temin, H. M. *J. Cell Physiol.* **69**, 377 (1967).

511. Temin, H. M. In: *Growth Regulating Substances for Animal Cells in Culture* (V. Defendi and M. Stoker, eds.) p. 103. Wistar Inst. Press, Philadelphia, 1967.

512. Temin, H. M., and Rubin, H. *Virology* **6**, 669 (1958).

513. Thompson, L. R., and McCarthy, B. J. *Biochem. Biophys. Research Commun.* **30**, 166 (1968).

514. Tiedemann, H. *Naturwissenschaften* **46**, 613 (1959).

515. Tiedemann, H., and Tiedemann, H. *Rev. Suisse Zool.* **71**, 117 (1964).

516. Tjio, J. H., Carbone, P. P., Whang, J., and Frei, E., III. *J. Nat. Cancer Inst.* **36**, 567 (1966).

517. Todaro, G. J., and Green, H. *Proc. Nat. Acad. Sci. U. S.* **55**, 302 (1966).

518. Todaro, G. J., Green, H., and Swift, M. R. *Science* **153**, 1252 (1966).

519. Todaro, G. J., Lazar, G. K., and Green, H. *J. Cell. Comp. Physiol.* **66**, 325 (1965).

520. Toivonen, S. *Rev. Suisse Zool.* **57**, 41 (1950).

521. Toivonen, S., Saxén, L., and Vainio, T. *Experientia* **17**, 86 (1961).

522. Trainin, N., Kaye, A. M., and Berenblum, I. *Biochem. Pharmacol.* **13**, 263 (1964).

523. Trentin J. J., Yabe, Y., and Taylor, G. *Science* **137**, 835 (1962).

524. Ursprung, H. *Arch. Entwicklungsmech. Organismen* **151**, 504 (1959).

525. Vasil, V., and Hildebrandt, A. C. *Science* **150**, 889 (1965).

526. Vendrely, R., and Sarciron, R. *Bull. Soc. Chimie Biol.* **26**, 214 (1944).

527. Vendrely, R., and Vendrely, C. *Experientia* **4**, 434 (1948).

528. Vigier, P., and Goldé, A. *C. r. Acad. Sci., Paris* **258**, 389 (1964).

198 *References*

529. Virchow, R. *Die krankhaften Geschwülste.* A. Hirschwald, Berlin, 1863.
530. Virchow, R. *Arch. path. Anat. Physiol.* **113**, 361 (1888).
531. Visfeldt, J. *Acta Pathol. Microbiol. Scand.* **58**, 414 (1963).
532. Vogt, P. K. *Proc. Nat. Acad. Sci. U. S.* **58**, 801 (1967).
533. Waddington, C. H. *Nature* **135**, 606 (1935).
534. Waddington, C. H. *Principles of Embryology.* 510 pp. George Allen and Unwin, London, 1956.
535. Waddington, C. H. *Principles of Development and Differentiation.* 115 pp. Macmillan, New York; and Collier-Macmillan, London, 1966.
536. Wald, N., Upton, A. C., Jenkins, V. K., and Borges, W. H. *Science* **143**, 810 (1964).
537. Waldeyer, H. W. G. *Arch. path. Anat. Physiol.* **41**, 470 (1867).
538. Waldeyer, H. W. G. *Arch. path. Anat. Physiol.* **55**, 67 (1872).
539. Wallace, R. E., Orsi, E. V., Ritter, H. B., and Moyer, A. W. *Exp. Cell Research* **25**, 671 (1961).
540. Warburg, O. *Biochem. Zeitschr.* **142**, 317 (1923).
541. Watkins, J. F., and Dulbecco, R. *Proc. Nat. Acad. Sci. U. S.* **58**, 1396 (1967).
542. Webster's International Unabridged Dictionary. 3rd ed. G. and C. Merriam, Springfield, Mass., 1961.
543. Wehr. *Arch. klin. Chirurgie* **39**, 226 (1889).
544. Weinhouse, S. *Science* **124**, 267 (1956); and: *Enzymes in Health and Disease* (D. M. Greenberg and H. A. Harper, eds.) p. 191. 1960.
545. Weiss, P. *The Principles of Development; A Text in Experimental Embryology.* 601 pp. H. Holt, New York, 1939.
546. Weiss, P. *Anat. Record* **88**, 205 (1944).
547. Weiss, P., and James, R. *Exp. Cell Research Suppl.* **3**, 381 (1955).
548. Weiss, P., and Wang, H. *Proc. Soc. Exp. Biol. Med.* **58**, 273 (1945).
549. Went, H. A. *J. Biophys. Biochem. Cytology* **5**, 353 (1959).
550. Went, H. A. *J. Biophys. Biochem. Cytology* **6**, 447 (1959).
551. Went, H. A., and Mazia, D. *Exp. Cell Research Suppl.* **7**, 200 (1959).
552. Westphal, H., and Dulbecco, R. *Proc. Nat. Acad. Sci. U. S.* **59**, 1158 (1968).
553. Wettstein, F. O., and Noll, H. *J. Mol. Biol.* **11**, 35 (1965).
554. White, P. R. *Bull. Torrey Botan. Club* **66**, 507 (1939).
555. White, P. R., and Braun, A. C. *Cancer Research* **2**, 597 (1942).
556. Wieland, H., and Dane, E. *Ztschr. physiol. Chemie* **219**, 240 (1933).
557. Wilkie, D. *The Cytoplasm in Heredity.* 115 pp. Methuen, London, 1964.
558. Willis, R. A. *The Spread of Tumours in the Human Body.* 540 pp. J. & A. Churchill, London, 1934.
559. Willis, R. A. *Pathology of Tumours.* 2nd ed. Mosby, St. Louis, Mo., 1953.

560. Willis, R. A. *The Borderland of Embryology and Pathology.* Chapter 14, p. 506, "Metaplasia." Butterworth, London, 1958.

561. Willmer, E. N. *J. Embryol. Exp. Morphol.* 6, 187 (1958).

562. Willmer, E. N. *Biol. Rev. Cambridge Philos. Soc.* 36, 368 (1961).

563. Witschi, E. *Verhandl. Naturforsch. Ges. Basel* 34, 33 (1922).

564. Witschi, E. *Arch. Entwicklungsmech. Organismen* 102, 168 (1924).

565. Witschi, E. *Proc. Soc. Exp. Biol. Med.* 27, 475 (1930).

566. Witschi, E. *Proc. Soc. Exp. Biol. Med.* 31, 419 (1934).

567. Witschi, E. *Cancer Research* 12, 763 (1952).

567a. Wolff, E. In: *Cell Differentiation and Morphogenesis.* International Lecture Course, Wageningen, The Netherlands, April 26–29, 1965. p. 1. North-Holland Publ., Amsterdam, 1966.

568. Wolff, E., and Ginglinger, A. *C. r. Acad. Sci., Paris* 200, 2118 (1935).

569. Wood, H. N. *Colloques Internat. Centre National de la Recherche Scient.,* No. 123, p. 97. Paris, 1964.

570. Wood, H. N., and Braun, A. C. *Proc. Nat. Acad. Sci. U. S.* 47, 1907 (1961).

571. Wood, H. N., and Braun, A. C. *Proc. Nat. Acad. Sci. U. S.* 54, 1532 (1965).

572. Wood, H. N., and Braun, A. C. *Ann. New York Acad. Sci.* 144, 244 (1967).

573. Woolley, G. W. In: *Physiopathology of Cancer* (F. Homburger and W. H. Fishman, eds.) Cassell, London, 1953.

574. Wyss, M. O. *Beitr. klin. Chirurgie* 49, 185 (1906).

575. Yamada, T. *Advances in Morphogenesis* 1, 1 (1961).

576. Yamagiwa, K., and Ichikawa, K. *J. Cancer Research* 3, 1 (1918).

577. Yerganian, G., Shein, H. M., and Enders, J. F. *Cytogenetics* 1, 314 (1962).

INDEX

Acetabularia, 164

Actinomycin D, 35, 36, 109, 114, 174

Activation of biosynthetic systems: in plant tumor cells, 55–63, 65–66; in animal tumor cells, 64–65, 97

Adenoviruses, oncogenic, 16, 86, 94

Adhesiveness of cells: shifting patterns, 66; in oncogenesis, 69

Adrenalin, 48, 54, 163

Agrobacterium tumefaciens, 9: thermal destruction of, 9; tumor-inducing principle, 9; transformation by, 9; *see also* Crown gall disease

Alkaline phosphatase, *see* Chronic myelocytic leukemia

Amoeba, 40, 42: *Amoeba proteus,* 37; *Pelomyxa carolinensis,* 44

Amphibians, reversal of tumor growth in, 142, 143, 144

Anaplasia, 29

Anchorage dependence, 93

Aneuploidy, 79, 81, 107, 134, 179; *see also* Chromosome changes

Anomalous differentiation and development, 3, 30, 129–32; relation to the tumor problem, 129, 153; progression of: identical twins, conjoined twins, double monsters, parasitic fetus (epignathus), ovarian dermoid teratoma (benign), teratocarcinoma (malignant), conventional tumors (benign and malignant), 129; experimental production of, 131, 132

Antichalone, 48

Anticodon, 165

Antigens: from sea urchin eggs, 43; relation to competence, 122; tissue-specific, 124; in tumors: 11, 16, 64, 71, 90, 93, 95, 155; viral-coded: T (tumor) antigen, 93, 95, 96, 155; coat antigen, 95; in Rous-sarcoma-transformed mammalian cells, 90; transplantation antigen, 95

L-Asparaginase, 86

Autonomous growth, 52–74: development of concept, 52–53; persistent activation of biosynthetic systems resulting in new pattern of synthesis: in animal tumors, 53–55, 64–65, 66–72; physiological basis in plant tumors (crown gall), 55–63, 65–66, 72–74; physiological basis in two other plant tumor systems, 62, 65; plant tumors as a model for an understanding of, 65–66; nutritional concept of autonomy, 59, 65; relevance to the tumor problem, 161–63

Autonomy, 5, 26–30; defined, 26–27

Auxins: as regulators of cell division in plants, 45, 163; as cell enlargement factor in plants, 45, 55, 57, 59, 61, 91; synergistic effect with cytokinins in plants, 45, 55, 57, 61, 163; role in plant tumor growth, 55; role in morphogenesis, 120, 140